Linda Norlander, RN, BSN, MS

To Comfort Always

A Nurse's Guide to End-of-Life Care

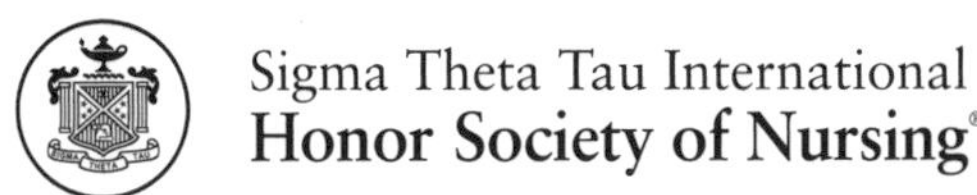

Sigma Theta Tau International
Honor Society of Nursing®

Sigma Theta Tau International

Acquisitions Editor: Cynthia Saver, RN, MS
Project Editor: Carla Hall
Copy Editor: Kevin Kent
Proofreader: Jackie Tirey

Cover Design by: Gary Adair
Interior Design and Page Composition by: Gary Adair

Printed in the United States of America
Printing and Binding by Printing Partners, Indianapolis, Indiana, USA

Sigma Theta Tau International
550 West North Street
Indianapolis, IN 46202

Visit our Web site at **www.nursingknowledge.org/STTI/books** for more information on our books.

ISBN-13: 978-1-930538-73-3
ISBN-10: 1-930538-73-1

Library of Congress Cataloging-in-Publication Data
Norlander, Linda, 1949-
To comfort always : a nurse's guide to end-of-life care / Linda Norlander.
p. ; cm.
Includes bibliographical references and index.
ISBN-13: 978-1-930538-73-3
ISBN-10: 1-930538-73-1
1. Terminal care. 2. Nursing. 3. Geriatric nursing. I. Sigma Theta Tau International. II. Title.
[DNLM: 1. Terminal Care--methods. 2. Nursing Care--methods. WY 152 N841t 2008]
RT87.T45N674 2009
616'.029--dc22

2008045865

First Printing
2008

Dedication

This book is written for all the nurses who have the courage and willingness to walk with patients on their final journeys. It is my hope that when you do this, you will be a full witness to the fundamental richness and grace of the human spirit.

Acknowledgements

I want to express my thanks and gratitude to the people who assisted me with this book. To Kerstin McSteen, RN, MS, ACHPN, who is a great hospice and palliative care nurse and a wonderful friend. To Jody Chrastek, RN, MS, for her guidance on care for children. To Mary Jo Tornberg, RN, MS, hospice clinical nurse specialist, who reviewed the book and provided expertise on updates and resources. To Greg Holmquist, PharmD, who provided updates on pain and symptom management. To Bree Norlander who helped with the formatting. And lastly, to Jerome Norlander who lived with the chaos of articles, texts, and drafts scattered all over the floor.

About the Author

Linda Norlander, RN, BSN, MS, is the manager of the Tacoma Group Health Home Care and Hospice program in Tacoma, Washington. She has written numerous journal articles on advance care planning, suffering at the end of life, and other hospice and end-of-life topics. Besides *To Comfort Always*, she co-wrote with Kerstin McSteen a book for baby boomers on how to talk about end-of-life decisions titled *Choices at the End of Life: Finding Out What Your Parents Want Before It's Too Late*. Linda has presented nationally on topics ranging from suffering at the end of life and advance care planning to statewide policy on aging. She has also conducted workshops for nurses on writing. She is a Robert Wood Johnson Executive Nurse Fellow.

Table of Contents

Dedication iii

Acknowledgements iv

About the Author v

Introduction x

Chapter 1 Where to Begin

Introduction 1

Guiding Principles of End of Life Care 2

Core Nursing Responsibilities: Skilled Clinician, Advocate, and Guide 4

What Do Patients and Families Want for Care at the End of Life? 5

When Do We Start Providing End of Life Care? 6

A Team Approach 7

Chapter 2 Advance Care Planning

The Courageous Conversation 11

Skilled Clinician: Understanding the Elements of Advance Care Planning 12

Advance Directives 15

A Note on DNR/DNI Status and POLST Forms 16

Advocating in Advance Care Planning: Making Sure Wishes Are Honored 16

Guiding in Advance Care Planning: Recognizing the Common Barriers 17

Common Questions Patients Ask About Advance Directives 19

Cultural Considerations in Advance Care Planning 20

Chapter 3 Pain Management: It's More Than Knowing the Meds

Listening to the Patient's Pain 23

Skilled Clinician: Assessment and Management of Pain 25

Advocating: Ensuring That the Patient's Pain Relief Goals Are Met 29

Guiding Patients and Families: Addressing Common Fears 31

Know the Resources 33

Chapter 4 Physical Symptom Management

Common Symptoms 35

Skilled Clinician: Assessment and Management of Common Symptoms 36

Advocating: Linking the Needs of the Patient and Family to the Health Care System 43

Guiding Patients and Families: Preparing, Listening, and Assuring 44

Chapter 5 Suffering: It's Not Just the Pain

What Is Suffering at the End of Life? 47

Skilled Clinician: Assessing Suffering 48

Advocating for Patients: Ensuring a Holistic View 52

Guiding Patients and Families: Start with Yourself 53

Chapter 6 Active Dying: The Final Days and Hours

Active Dying: What Does It Mean? 57

Skilled Clinician: Assessing and Intervening When Death Is Near 58

Advocating for Both the Patient and Family: Communication Is the Key 63

Guiding: Walking That Difficult Path 64

A Note on Withdrawing Life-Sustaining or Life-Extending Treatment 65

Chapter 7 After the Death: The Long Journey to the Car

What Happens after a Patient Dies? 67

Skilled Clinician: Understanding Grief 68

Advocating for the Family: Accommodating Their Comfort Needs 69

Guiding the Family: Accepting the Loss 70

Self Care 73

Chapter 8 When a Child Is Dying: Pediatric End of Life

Children Die, Too ... 75

Skilled Clinician: Assessing and Intervening in the Care of Children ... 77

Advocating for Children: Meeting the Needs of Both the Patient and the Family ... 80

Guiding Children and Families: Understanding the Needs of the Child ... 82

Chapter 9 Cultural Sensitivity: Looking through Different Eyes

Making Room for Cultural Diversity ... 85

Understand Your Own Beliefs ... 87

Listen to the Patients ... 88

Avoid Stereotyping and Making Assumptions ... 89

Use Trained Medical Interpreters ... 89

Use Community Resources ... 90

Advocating for Patients and Families ... 91

Chapter 10 Hospice

A Philosophy of Care ... 95

Who Qualifies for Hospice Care? ... 96

How Do I Approach Patients and Families about Hospice Care? ... 97

The Hospice Medicare Benefit ... 98

Advocating for Your Patients ... 100

Chapter 11 Ethical Issues in End-of-Life Care

Health Care Ethics ... 104

Common Ethical Dilemmas and Conflicts ... 105

Role of the Skilled Clinician in Difficult Decisions ... 106

Advocate: Making Sure Wishes Are Honored ... 107

Guide ... 108

What about a Nurse's Personal Ethics, Beliefs, and Values? ... 109

Ethics and Culture ... 109

Chapter 12 A Final Note: Taking Care
Burning Brightly, Burning Dimly 113
Living in the Present Moment 114
The Joy and the Laughter 115
A Final Note 115

Index 117

Introduction

I Didn't Know What I Didn't Know

Thirty years ago when I was a novice home care nurse, I was assigned to Margaret, a 70-year-old woman with terminal liver cancer. She lived with her husband and a disabled son. For five months, I struggled in vain to make her comfortable, to control her pain, to relieve her physical symptoms. I watched her diminish in front of me, her skin breaking down, her eyes glazed with pain, and I felt a growing helplessness. Looking back, I know she sensed my helplessness. I remember walking into her bedroom one day with dread. She was comfortable only in the fetal position on her left side. It was agony for her to be moved. Her husband's eyes said, "Do something." In desperation, I held her and asked, "Is there something more I can do for you?"

"No," she whispered.

I didn't believe her.

Back then, *I didn't know what I didn't know*. I didn't know that her pain and symptoms could be managed, that dying is multilayered and multidimensional, and that Margaret's personal, family, and spiritual suffering could be addressed. I didn't know the crucial role that nursing could have played in helping Margaret die peacefully and comfortably. I wasn't truly present for Margaret or her family.

Fortunately, much has changed since the days that I struggled to care for her. Hospice has emerged as a gold standard of care for those who are dying. Research and education focused on how to best care for those at the end of life has grown. Yet, we still have a long way to go to make sure that patients like Margaret get the right kind of nursing care.

This book is a primer for nurses in end-of-life care. It is not meant to be a comprehensive text or an all-inclusive manual. Rather, it is meant to educate nurses enough so they know what they don't know and know where to find the appropriate tools and resources. (See "Suggested Resources" at the end of the Introduction.)

Three Nursing Roles

Most of the chapters have the nursing role divided into three parts:

1. The nurse as a skilled clinician,
2. The nurse as an advocate, and
3. The nurse as a guide.

Skilled Clinician: This refers to the assessment and technical skills needed to manage care for someone at the end of his or her life. If I'd had the clinical skills to care for Margaret, I would have known how to assess her pain, how to use other health care team members as resources, and how to intervene to keep her comfortable.

Advocate: This refers to the work a nurse needs to do to obtain the best care for a patient. If I'd had advocacy skills, I would have insisted on better pain relief from Margaret's doctor. I would have looked at my home care agency and worked on ensuring social work availability for Margaret's family and clear systems for reaching a nurse on call.

Guide: This refers to the knowledge, communication, and intuition a nurse needs in order to walk with a patient during that difficult last journey. If I had been a skilled guide for Margaret, I would have been better able to prepare her for her death, better able to help her husband with simple assurances, and I would have been there for her husband and son's walk into bereavement.

Linda Norlander, RN, BSN, MS

Suggested Resources

Books

A comprehensive nursing textbook on end-of-life care:

Ferrell, B.R., & Coyle, N. (Eds.). (2005). Textbook of palliative nursing (2nd ed.). New York: Oxford University Press.

A book that blends the clinical, psycho-social, ethical, and spiritual role the nurse assumes in caring for dying patients.

Matzo, M.L., & Sherman, D.W. (Eds.). (2005). Palliative care nursing: Quality care to the end of life (2nd ed.). New York: Springer.

A systematic exploration of the foundations needed to provide the best care for patients.

Zerwekh, J.V. (2006). Nursing care at the end of life: Palliative care for patients and families. Philadelphia: F.A. Davis.

Web Resources

End-of-Life Nursing Education Consortium (ELNEC), a national initiative to improve end-of-life care. www.aacn.nche.edu/ELNEC/

EPERC is the medical educator resource for peer-reviewed end-of-life teaching materials. Also search for recommended books and articles. http://www.eperc.mcw.edu/

Hospice and Palliative Nurses Association. Information about membership, publications, conferences, and certification. www.hpna.org/

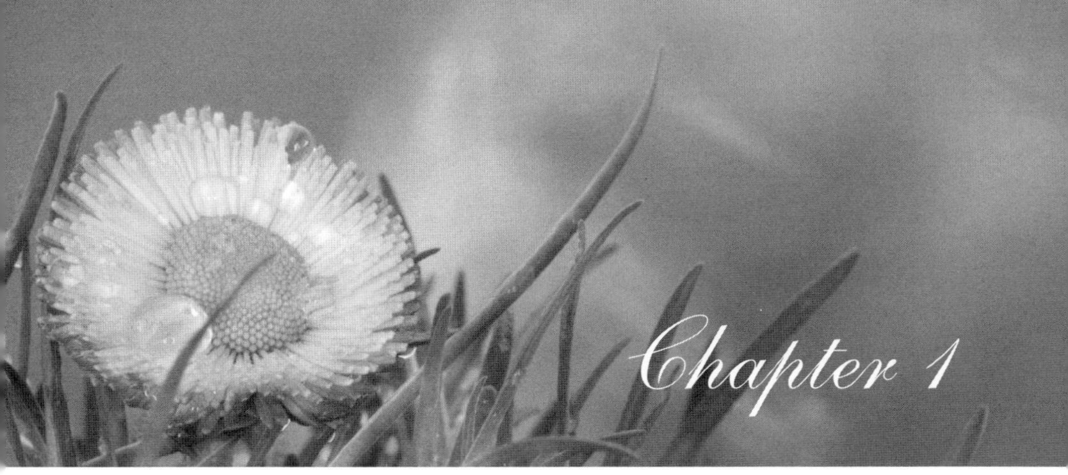

Where to Begin

Death is not a medical event. It is a personal and family story of profound choices, of momentous words, and telling silences.

—Steve Miles, M.D.

Introduction

Greg is 46 years old. He was diagnosed 7 months ago with non-small cell lung cancer. He has gone through a course of chemotherapy and radiation treatments. His oncologist has just told him that the tumor in his lung is growing and that he has few treatment options left. His oncology nurse is part of the conversation. When the doctor leaves, Greg turns to her and asks, "Does this mean I'm dying? What am I supposed to do now?"

The nurse sits quietly with him for a few moments before replying, "I want you to know that we will stay with you through this."

Greg has reached a point in his illness where a cure is no longer possible. Compassionate and comprehensive nursing care can ensure that his needs are met during his life's final journey. His oncology nurse has begun this care by listening to him and assuring him that he won't be abandoned. One of her next steps will include helping him discuss his care wishes and goals.

Guiding Principles of End of Life Care

While death has remained a constant over the course of history, the process of dying has changed over the past 100 years. Medical advances have changed death from a sudden event into an often long journey with many events. We have increased the life span, created complex medical choices, and shaped a new population of people with chronic illnesses.

We have not done well, however, in providing care at the end of life. Classic studies conducted in the 1990s highlighted concerns regarding health care at the end of life. These reports chronicled poor pain control and suffering in those who were dying, lack of family inclusion in care and other decision making, and inconsistent and conflicting decision making by the health care system (SUPPORT, 1995).

While nursing has been on the forefront of many advances in end-of-life care including pain and symptom management, nurses continue to be challenged because we often work in environments (hospitals and skilled nursing facilities) where the focus is on maintaining the functions of physiological systems rather than on the patient as a whole being. (Zerwekh, 2006.) With this emphasis, many nurses lack the skills, training, or experience needed to address the complexity of care required by a dying patient.

According to the American Association of Colleges of Nurses (AACN)

> People in our country deny death, believing that medical science can cure any patient. Death often is seen as a failure of the health care system rather than a natural aspect of life. This belief affects all health professionals, including nurses. Despite their undisputed technical and interpersonal skills, professional nurses may not be completely comfortable with the specialized knowledge and skills needed to provide quality end-of-life care to patients. (AACN, Fact Sheet, paragraph 4. 2008)

To help patients like Greg, nurses need to understand the concepts and components of end-of-life care and be skilled practitioners of the nursing arts.

First and foremost, end-of-life care is patient goal centered and should be provided for those who have a limited life expectancy. The term *palliative care* is often used when discussing end-of-life care. The word *palliative* means to abate or reduce the intensity. The concept of palliative care is based on the provision of comfort and relief, rather than that of cure.

According to the World Health Organization, palliative care "improves the quality of life of patients and families who face life-threatening illness by providing pain and symptom relief, spiritual and psychosocial support from diagnosis to end of life bereavement" (WHO, 2008, paragraph 3).

Hospice care is often looked at as a subset of palliative care focused on those patients who are no longer seeking active, curative treatment and who have a life expectancy of 6 months or less. The best end-of-life care encompasses a holistic approach that recognizes the physical, personal, family, and spiritual realms of the patient. The patient's family should always be considered part of the unit of care. The National Hospice and Palliative Care Organization states in its preamble to standards of practice:

> Hospice affirms the concept of palliative care as an intensive program that enhances comfort and promotes the quality of life for individuals and their families. When cure is no longer possible, hospice recognizes that a peaceful and comfortable death is an essential goal of health care. Hospice believes that death is an integral part of the life cycle and that intensive palliative care focuses on pain relief, comfort, and enhanced quality of life as appropriate goals for the terminally ill. Hospice also recognizes the potential for growth that often exists within the dying experience for the individual and his/her family and seeks to protect and nurture this potential (National Hospice Palliative Care Organization, 2008, paragraph 1).

Five guiding principles for end-of-life care can help nurses frame a comprehensive and compassionate plan for patients and families. (See the sidebar, "Guiding Principles for Comprehensive End-of-Life Nursing Care.")

Guiding Principles for Comprehensive End-of-Life Nursing Care

1. **Patient and family preference for treatment and care will be discussed and respected.** Nurses will ask about patient and family goals and preferences, include patient and family in the decision process, provide assistance and resources to formulate advance care plans, and honor written health care directives.
2. **Undesirable symptoms will be relieved.** Nurses will believe reports of distress, do their best to relieve all undesirable

symptoms, anticipate and prevent undesirable symptoms when possible, and provide urgent treatment of severe symptoms.

3. **Emotional, spiritual, and personal suffering will be addressed.** Nurses will ask about emotional, spiritual, and personal suffering and offer the help of interdisciplinary or community resources.
4. **Patients will be prepared for their death, and families will be prepared for the death of their loved one.** Nurses will provide honest information on what is likely to happen and provide guidance in planning how to handle predictable events.
5. **Grieving will be acknowledged.** Nurses will provide a quiet and safe place for families to grieve, accommodate family wishes to be with the deceased loved one, and acknowledge that grieving is a long-term process.

These principles were adapted from recommendations by the Minnesota Commission on End of Life Care (Hospice Minnesota, 2002).

Core Nursing Responsibilities: Skilled Clinician, Advocate, and Guide

Ten years ago, 22-year-old Jennifer's father was dying of leukemia in a busy public hospital. She sat with him alone, the only family member at the bedside. The nursing staff avoided his room. Jennifer agonized with every breath her father took, interpreting his gasping as a struggle. Finally, in desperation to give him relief, she took off his oxygen mask. To her horror, her father stopped breathing. She blamed herself for his death. No one sat with her or explained to her what those final moments would look like. She held onto this secret for years until she finally confessed to a friend who was a hospice nurse, "I think I killed my Dad." Her nurse friend assured her that she was not responsible for her father's death and that she gave him a precious gift by being at his side when he died. On hearing this, Jennifer began to cry. "I've carried this all these years. You mean I didn't kill him?"

Years of guilt and suffering could have been averted by a competent and compassionate nurse at the time Jennifer's father was dying. Three core competencies are critical for end-of-life care:

1. A *skilled clinician* who understands end-of-life symptom management and can provide the best comfort care.
2. An *advocate* who can ensure that all members of the health care team are available.
3. A *guide* who can walk with patients and their families through the dying experience.

What Do Patients and Families Want for Care at the End of Life?

The first step for a nurse in becoming a skilled clinician, an advocate, and a guide is a clear understanding of what patients and families want for care at the end of life. Knops, Srinivasan, & Meyers (2005) reviewed research articles focused on patient preferences at the end of life. They found that preferences can evolve as the disease progresses, that patients want a sense of control over the disease, control over suffering, and control over death itself. The key desires of patients and families at the end of life are process-oriented and relationship-based rather than focused on medical goals (Steinhauser et. al., 2000). Additionally, patients prefer to die at home (Tang, 2003).

Several themes emerge when looking at patient and family preferences:

- **Pain and symptom management:** Patients want assurances that physical discomfort will be relieved.
- **Family involvement:** Patients want their families involved in decision making and in care.
- **Care at home:** When asked, most patients express a desire to receive their end-of-life care at home.
- **Preparation for death:** Patients want to know what will happen as they near death.
- **Completion:** Patients want the opportunity to say good-bye and leave some kind of legacy.
- **Affirmation of the whole person:** Patients want to be recognized as still having something to contribute. They want to be a person first, then a person who is dying.

When Do We Start Providing End of Life Care?

The shift from a focus on curative care to a focus on palliative and end-of-life care does not usually begin with a sudden event. For most patients who are nearing the end of life, the journey has been long—sometimes years. Patients describe a roller-coaster ride with periods of very good times and periods of very low times. Often as they ride the roller coaster, they experience some type of incremental decline. Good palliative and end-of-life care is often delayed because of the failure to recognize changes in the patient's condition. Look for indicators that signal the need to begin discussing end-of-life care. (See the sidebar, "Red Flags.")

A good nursing assessment involves careful attention to the whole person. Ask these questions:

1. Has the patient changed?
2. How was the patient six months ago? Three months ago? Two weeks ago?
3. Has the patient lost weight?
4. Is he or she less energetic, less able to do everyday activities?
5. Does the patient have increased symptomology?
6. Does the patient experience dyspnea, fatigue, or pain?
7. Has the family seen a change in the last six months? Three months? Two weeks?

After a patient has been determined to be at risk for dying, the change from curative to a palliative focus of care still might be gradual. For some patients this shift might never occur. Nurses who advocate for patients and help guide them have a responsibility to help facilitate ongoing discussions with the patients about their care wishes and goals. No matter what setting you practice in—hospital, long-term care facility, clinic, or home—it is of utmost importance to attend to the patient's comfort needs as the patient sees them.

Red Flags

The following are red flags that can signal the need to begin discussing end-of-life care (Norlander & McSteen, 2000):

- Illnesses or conditions that could be considered potentially life-threatening or life-limiting.
- A change in functional status with dependencies in two or more activities of daily living.
- Repeat hospitalizations and emergency room visits.
- Anyone for whom you would answer "yes" to the question: "Would you be surprised if this person were alive in one to two years?"

A Team Approach

The needs of patients and families at the end of life are multidimensional. As a nurse, you have a large toolbox of skills ranging from clinical and technical skills to assessment and communication skills. However, in caring for dying patients and their families, you need to recognize that you cannot do it all. A good clinician draws on the expertise of other professionals to enhance practice and provide the highest level of care.

For example, Steinhauser et al. (2000) identified dying patients' needs to achieve spiritual peace. The patient might best accomplish this with assistance from a chaplain, community clergy, or a counselor. Referring patients to other professional resources can be as important to a patient's comfort as administering the most appropriate dose of morphine. You can use a wide variety of professional team members when caring for patients at the end of life.

Physician

The role of the physician in the care of dying patients cannot be overstressed. Not only do physicians direct clinical care, but they have the expertise in disease pathology. Most importantly, patients and families often look to the physician for guidance during these difficult times. Because of this important relationship, nurses need to work in partnership with physicians in providing the best care for patients and families.

Social Worker

Social workers are skilled in communication and group facilitation and are knowledgeable about community resources. They can be critical in helping patients with long-term planning, in helping to facilitate family discussions, and in counseling patients and families.

Chaplain or Spiritual Care Worker

Many of the issues that patients and families deal with during life's final journey revolve around spiritual and religious matters. Treatment decisions are sometimes based on religious beliefs. This is often a time for self-reflection and contemplation. Patients may need help articulating and thinking through some of the basic questions of life, such as "What am I here for?" Often hospital and long-term care facility chaplains as well as community spiritual leaders can be of help.

Pharmacist

A wide array of pharmacological treatments exist for pain and symptom control. The pharmacist has expertise in available medications, drug interactions, optimal delivery methods, and indications for use.

Dietician

Patients and families often struggle with nutrition and hydration issues. Dieticians can counsel on types of foods to prepare, supplements, and feeding methods.

Other Team Members

Other team members may include physical, occupational, and speech therapists, as well as psychologists, volunteers, and clinical nurse specialists. The best nursing care at the end of life is provided in a team atmosphere. Beware of feeling as though you have to be all things to all patients.

Summary

Comprehensive nursing care for patients at the end of life can only be provided using a holistic approach. The five guiding principles of end-of-life care can provide a framework for that care. You need to discuss goals and wishes with patients and family. You must take care to address the physical, personal, family, and spiritual needs of the patient. The best care is provided in an interprofessional team environment. Your nursing role includes being a skilled clinician, advocate, and guide.

References

American Association of Colleges of Nursing (AACN). End of life nursing consortium fact sheet. Retrieved 4 October 2008 from http://www.aacn.nche.edu/ELNEC/factsheet.htm

Knops, K.M., Srinivasan, M., & Meyers, F.J. (Dec. 2005). Patient desires: a model for assessment of patient preferences for care of severe or terminal illness. *Palliative and Supportive Care*; 3(4): 289-99.

Hospice Minnesota. (2002). Minnesota Commission on End of Life Care Report. Retrieved 11 June 2008 from www.hospicemn.org

National Hospice and Palliative Care Organization. (2008). Preamble to NHPCO standards of practice. Retrieved 4 October 2008 from http://www.nhpco.org/i4a/pages/Index.cfm?pageID=5308

Norlander, L., & McSteen, K. (2000). The kitchen table discussion: A creative way to discuss end-of-life issues. *Home Healthcare Nurse* 18(8): 532–539.

Steinhauser, K.E., Clipp, E.C., McNeilly, M., Christakis, N.A., McIntyre, L.M., & Tulsky, J.A. (2000). In search of a good death: Observations of patient, families and providers. *Annals of Internal Medicine* 132(10): 825–832.

SUPPORT Principal Investigators. (1995). A controlled trial to improve care for seriously ill hospitalized patients. *Journal of the American Medical Association*. 274: 1591–1598.

Tang, S.T. (2003). When death is imminent: Where terminally ill patients with cancer prefer to die and why. *Cancer Nursing* 26(3):245-251.

World Health Organization. Palliative care. Retrieved 1 April 2008 from http://www.who.int/cancer/palliative/en/

Zerwekh, J.V. (2006). *Nursing care at the end of life: Palliative care for patients and families*. Philadelphia: FA Davis.

Other Resources

National Consensus Project for Quality End of Life Care. www.nationalconsensusproject.org

National Hospice and Palliative Care Organization. www.nhpco.org

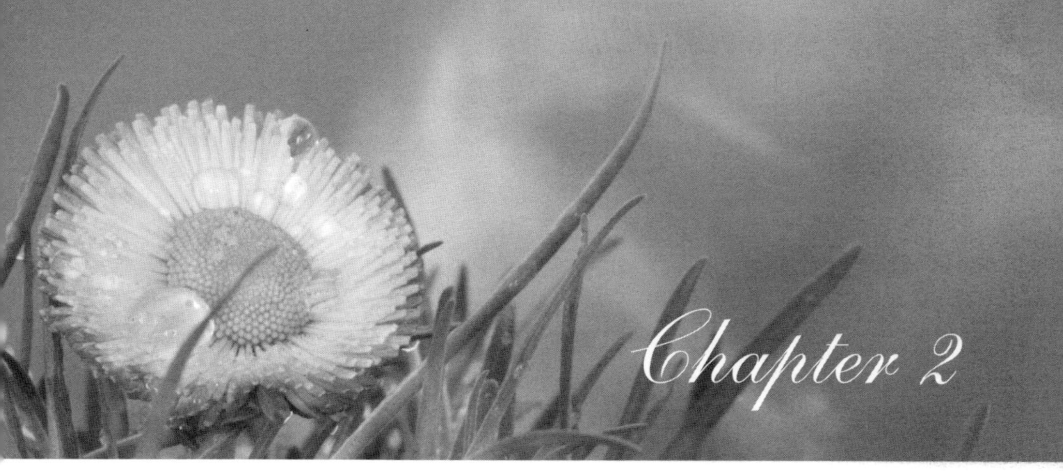

Advance Care Planning

It's always a little tough to talk about one's own mortality, but I've come to grips with it. After all, I've been at death's door three times now.

—Home-care patient discussing advance care planning

The Courageous Conversation

Stephanie is a 62-year-old divorced woman with 2 children and 3 grandchildren. She was diagnosed with ALS (amyotrophic lateral sclerosis) 4 months ago. Since her diagnosis, she has experienced increased lower extremity weakness. She fell 3 days ago, suffering a soft tissue knee injury and fracturing her right wrist. She is hospitalized for surgery to stabilize the wrist. When the nurse comes in to care for her, Stephanie starts to cry. "How am I going to go home like this? What happens if I get worse? I've heard that some people go on breathing machines. I'm not sure I want that."

The nurse asks, "Have you talked with your doctor about what you might see with this illness?"

Stephanie says, "No. I've been waiting for her to bring it up."

The nurse sits by the bedside with Stephanie and says, "I'd like to spend a few minutes with you. Can we talk about some of these things?"

Stephanie's nurse is embarking on a difficult and courageous conversation. This talk is the beginning of advance care planning for Stephanie. These discussions are not easy for either the patient and family or the nurse because we live in a society that is not comfortable talking about dying. The National Hospice Foundation conducted a poll and found that people in the baby boom generation (born between 1946 and 1964) are more comfortable talking with their children about safe sex than they are talking with their terminally ill parents about death (National Hospice Foundation, 1999). As nurses, we have not been trained to have these conversations. Yet, too often the critical end-of-life care discussions are delayed until a patient is in crisis or too close to death to participate (Hume, 1998; Wilkinson, Wenger, & Shugarman, 2007). Earlier identification of patient wishes can prevent inappropriate and often unwanted treatments.

Skilled Clinician: Understanding the Elements of Advance Care Planning

Clinical nursing skills in working with patients at the end of life include knowledge and understanding of advance care planning. If you know and understand the key elements in the advance care planning discussion about end-of-life care goals, you can facilitate a therapeutic interaction. (See the sidebar "Key Elements of Advance Care Planning Discussion.")

Advance care planning is a thoughtful, facilitated discussion that encompasses a lifetime of values, beliefs, and goals for the patient and family. It is not merely a discussion of medical treatment choices. People make decisions throughout life based on their experiences, values, goals, and socio-cultural norms, and making decisions about how they would like to be treated at the end of life is no different. Completion of an advance directive (also known as a living will or health care directive) can be part of advance care planning, but this is only one component in a much larger discussion.

People who are significant to the patient, such as family, friends, and caregivers, should be invited to participate in the advance care planning discussion as the patient wishes and allows. However, end-of-life issues might be a topic that patients and their loved ones, in an effort to protect each other, find difficult to discuss openly. As an objective, skilled clinician, you can help guide these discussions and clarify thoughts and feelings that the patient and family have.

Any advance care planning discussion should be held in a setting that is comfortable for the patient and family. One of the most effective places to have this discussion is in the patient's home. As a nurse working in institutional settings, you cannot always gather a patient and family "around the kitchen table." However, you can strive to make the setting as comfortable and informal as possible. Is it private and free from distraction? Are the chairs comfortable? A cramped examination room, for example, is not the best place for initiating such important and vital communication.

Key Elements of Advance Care Planning Discussion

Helping a patient and family talk about end-of-life wishes and goals involves understanding some key elements of the discussion (Norlander & McSteen, 2000):

- Patient goals and values
- Patient experience with death
- Patient understanding of illness
- Family support and understanding of patient goals and values
- Communication with physician
- Resources

Patient Goals and Values

Advance care planning is an opportunity for a respectful, therapeutic discussion with patients as they think about how they want to die. Patient goals and values are at the heart of any advance care planning discussion. Some patients value living a long life, living an active life, or enjoying the company of friends. Others place financial concerns as a top priority. Goals can be very broad or very specific. One patient expressed the goal that she wanted to live long enough to see the birth of a grandchild. Another wanted to make sure he could leave a financial legacy for his children. An important question you can ask regarding care goals is, "What do you hope for?"

Patients also often have a strong preference for where they would like their care as they are dying. A 72-year-old widower said, "I grew up in this house. I've lived here all my life. This is what I know. I'd like to stay here until I die."

Patient Experience with Death

A patient's own experience with the death of a loved one can have a profound impact on care wishes at the end of life. For example, an 85-year-old patient with chronic heart failure expressed a great fear of dying in a long-term care facility. When the nurse explored this fear with her, she explained that her husband had died that way, and she didn't want her children to experience that again. In another case, a middle-aged man who as a child had witnessed his father's death expressed a fear of dying in extreme pain. You can ask the question, "What has it been like for others you've known when they died?"

Patient Understanding of Illness

You need to explore how patients understand the illness. Do they see it as life threatening? Are they expecting a cure or improvement? Do they understand their treatment choices? How patients view the illness can be very different from how the medical profession sees it or how the family understands it. At the beginning of one advance care planning discussion, a family specifically asked the social worker not to say anything about dying to the patient because he didn't know he was terminal and he might lose hope. To the family's surprise, when the social worker asked the patient his understanding of the illness, the patient said, "Well, it's pretty obvious, isn't it? I'm dying." A way you can find out what a patient knows is to say, "Tell me what you know about your illness," or to ask, "What has the doctor told you?"

Family Support of Patient Goals and Values

An effective advance care planning discussion must involve the patient's family. Discuss any conflict or disagreement with a patient's wishes. As one patient stated, "I'm glad we've discussed this because those decisions won't fall on the children now." This is an opportune time to name someone as the health care proxy, the spokesperson if the patient is unable to speak or make decisions.

Physician Communication

Patients look to their physicians for guidance during the course of a disease. You can help patients and families frame the questions to discuss with the doctor. You can also be invaluable in clarifying the patient and family understanding of what the physician has said.

Resources

A discussion of resources available to patients is an integral part of advance care planning. Many patients do not know that they have options that can help, options such as hospice, community senior services, and community church support. This discussion also provides the opportunity to help a patient fill out a health care directive to provide written documentation of care wishes. For example, after an advance care planning session, a patient requested extra brochures on hospice. "I'm going to show these to my doctor and tell him this is what I want when it's time."

Advance Directives

Advance directives are legally binding documents that direct health care and decision making when patients are no longer able to speak for themselves. Legislation on the use of advance directives and the form they must take varies from state to state.

Generally, two types of advance directives exist:

- **Living Will or Health Care Directive:** The living will is a document filled out by the patient with specific instructions on health care. It often addresses issues such as artificial nutrition and hydration and use of resuscitation and intubation.
- **Durable Health Care Power of Attorney, Health Care Agent, or Health Care Proxy:** With this document, patients can designate a specific person to speak for them if they are unable to speak for themselves.

A Note on DNR/DNI Status and POLST Forms

Patients and sometimes nurses become confused about the difference between a health care directive and a do not resuscitate/do not intubate (DNR/DNI) order. They are not the same. A health care directive is a legal document reflecting the *patient's* wishes for treatment at the end of life. A DNR/DNI is a *physician's* treatment order. DNR/DNI status written in a patient's medical record does not mean an advance care planning discussion has taken place.

Physician's Order for Life-Sustaining Treatment (POLST) forms are used in some states. This form expands on the DNR/DNI order to include other treatments such as antibiotics, hydration, and hospitalization. While it is still a physician's signed order, the POLST is generally filled out following discussion with the patient and family. More information on POLST can be found at http://www.ohsu.edu/ethics/polst/

Advocating in Advance Care Planning: Making Sure Wishes Are Honored

Nurses play a key role not only in initiating and facilitating discussion about end-of-life care, but also in making sure that these wishes are honored. You can advocate for your patients on several levels.

First, on the patient/family level, find out if the patient has an advance directive. If not, offer the resources to facilitate the discussion. Use the skills of other health care team members such as the social worker or chaplain. Engage the physician in the discussion by setting up a time the patient and family can talk with him or her about treatment preferences.

If the patient does have an advance directive, ask the important question, "Does this document reflect your current wishes?" Make sure that the patient and family understand what has been written. Also, make sure that the care orders reflect the patient's wishes. K.E. Covinsky, et al, (2000), reporting on the results of a large multihospital study in the *Journal of the American Geriatric Society*, notes that even when a written directive was in the chart, only 25 percent of the physicians were aware the directive existed.

In this study, patients with written advance directives were no more likely than patients without them to have their preferences for or against CPR honored. Patients and families sometimes assume that if choices are written down, they will be honored.

On an organizational level, ask these questions:

- Do you have a system for making sure that advance directives are honored? When a nurse in a Midwestern skilled nursing facility discovered that advance directives were ignored because they were "buried" in the back of the medical record, she changed the system to have a listing of treatment wishes placed in the Kardex.
- Do you have the option of support from a professional team such as an interdisciplinary ethics committee? If not, consider forming one.

Guiding in Advance Care Planning: Recognizing the Common Barriers

As discussed earlier in the chapter, this can be a difficult yet courageous conversation for the patient and family and the nurse. You face several challenges concerning this conversation, including how to approach the subject with patients and how to overcome common barriers to the discussion. (See the sidebar on "Helpful and Supportive Phrases.") Recognizing some of the common barriers to the discussion can help you as you sit down with the patient and family.

Helpful and Supportive Phrases

The following statements could be used to initiate the advance care planning discussion:

- "Have you thought about what kind of care you would want if you could no longer speak for yourself?"
- "Making decisions before a crisis is a gift you can give to your family."
- "Advance care planning gives you some control over your future."
- "This is an opportunity to develop a written health care directive."

Will the Patient Lose Hope If I Bring Up the Topic?

Many nurses fear that if they bring up the subject of end-of-life care wishes, the patient might lose hope. However, research has shown that the actual process of discussing end-of-life issues stimulates therapeutic conversations between patients and health care professionals, and it leaves patients and families with an increased sense of feeling cared for and understood (Miles, Koepp & Weber, 1996).

The most important need of patients and families is assurance that they are not going to be abandoned and that every effort is going to be made to optimize the highest quality of life in their remaining days. With this understanding, you can work with patients and families in determining goals for treatment at the end of life, and the patient and family can better trust that you are going to continue to support them in any situation.

Isn't Advance Care Planning the Physician's Responsibility?

The physician should be one of the health care team members involved in advance care planning. The physician might know more about prognosis and treatment of a particular diagnosis, but the nurse often has a much better perspective on how a patient is functioning. This is an opportunity for you to prepare patients and families for a discussion with the physician and also to empower them to state their care wishes and goals.

I'm Not Comfortable Talking about Death and Dying

You might find that in talking about advance care planning with patients, your own personal experiences and issues are brought to the surface. Your own personal history of loss and death can have a positive or negative impact on professional practice. You are encouraged to explore your own feelings, beliefs, and experiences. Completing a health care directive for yourself can be a helpful exercise and can improve your comfort level with the process.

Decision Making at the Time of a Crisis

Much as it would be nice to know a patient's care wishes at the end of life, advance care planning is often not done. If you work in an acute care setting, especially an intensive care unit or emergency department, you might be faced with distraught patients and families trying to make hard decisions about such aggressive treatments as resuscitation, intubation, artificial nutrition, hydration, and dialysis. In emotionally charged times such as these, your guidance with good communication and listening skills is essential.

- **Clarify choices in simple language**. Patients and families might not understand the word *intubation*, but they should understand the phrase "a tube that is placed in the windpipe and connected to a breathing machine."
- **Explore possible preferences with the family if the patient is unable to speak.** If the patient is unable to speak and does not have a health care directive or agent, ask the family if they can recall any conversations with the patient that would indicate the patient's wishes.
- **Clarify "benefit versus burden."** If a treatment is chosen, what are the benefits and what are the burdens associated with it? Will it make the patient more comfortable? Extend life? What kind of care is involved? What can be expected to happen in 2 days or 2 months?
- **Engage other team members.** Often, patient and families find comfort in talking with a chaplain or community clergy before making decisions.

Common Questions Patients Ask About Advance Directives

The advance directive document can be very confusing for patients and families. In your nursing role as a clinician, advocate, and guide, you will find it helpful to be prepared for some of the common questions patients and families have.

I already have a will. Why do I need to fill out one of these forms? Patients are often confused by the array of legal terminology and become mixed up between the words *will*, *living will*, *power of attorney*, and *health care power of attorney*. Reiterate to the patient that a will and a power of attorney both refer to financial and estate planning, not health care planning.

Do I need a lawyer to help me with an advance directive? *No.* Advance directives are health care decisions and can be filled out by the patient and family or with assistance from a nurse, physician, or other health care professional (Sabatino, 2008).

Whom should I name as my health care agent? You as a nurse can help facilitate the decision on whom the patient names as his or her agent (medical power of attorney or proxy) by asking the patient whom he or she trusts to carry out his or her wishes. The patient needs to discuss care wishes and goals with this person before naming him or her as the proxy.

Will my wishes be honored? In most states, health care professionals are legally bound to honor the patient's wishes. Sometimes this does not occur for several reasons:

- The advance directive is not available at the time treatment decisions need to be made. This is especially true in emergency situations.
- The advance directive is not clear. Statements such as *no heroic measures* can be interpreted in many different ways.
- The health care proxy is unsure of the patient's wishes.

Can I change my mind? Every patient has the right to change or revoke an advance directive. In fact, patients often rethink treatment decisions during the course of an illness. Review advance directives with patients on a periodic basis.

Cultural Considerations in Advance Care Planning

The cultural traditions of a patient and family need to be taken into consideration when talking about advance care planning and end-of-life goals. We need to recognize that in some communities families actively protect loved ones from the knowledge of the illness and from any talk about dying. In others, the decision-making is done by family members rather than the patient. (Wilkinson, Wenger, & Shugarman, 2007). It is important to be sensitive to different traditions and beliefs. When in doubt, ask, "How would you like us to discuss your illness and your care preferences?"

Summary

Advance care planning is much more than asking patients if they have a living will or if they want to be resuscitated. It's a comprehensive and therapeutic discussion of patients' values, care wishes, and goals at the end of life, and it is a vital component of holistic nursing practice for any patient with a life-limiting illness.

References

Covinsky, K.E., et al. (May 2000). Communication and decision-making in seriously ill patients: Findings of the SUPPORT project. *Journal of the American Geriatric Society.* 448(5 Suppl): S187-93.

Hume, M. (1998). Improving care at the end of life. *The Quality Letter for Health Care Leaders* 10:6.

Miles, S.H., Koepp, R., & Weber, E.P. (1996). Advance end-of-life treatment planning: A research review. *Archives of Internal Medicine* 156:1062–1068.

National Hospice Foundation. (1999). Survey, April 9–20. Washington, DC.

Norlander, L., & McSteen, K. (2000). The kitchen table discussion: A creative way to talk about advance care planning. *Home Healthcare Nurse* 18(8): 532–539.

Sabatino, C.P. (2008). 10 legal myths about advance medical directives. American Bar Association: Washington, DC. Retrieved 14 October 2008 from http://www.abanet.org/aging/publications/docs/10legalmythsarticle.pdf

Wilkinson, A., Wenger, N., & Shugarman, L.R. (2007). Literature review on advanced directives. U.S. Department of Health and Human Services, Office of Aging, Disability and Long Term Care Policy. Retrieved 14 October 2008 from http://aspe.hhs.gov/daltcp/reports/2007/advdirlr.pdf

Other Resources

Aging with Dignity Web site. Provides the health care directive document "Five Wishes," which is legal in 40 states and is also available in 20 languages. www.agingwithdignity.org

Caring Connections, supported by the National Hospice and Palliative Care Organization. Provides state-specific advance directive forms, as well as resources on advance care planning and end-of-life care. http://caringinfo.org

The Do-Not-Resuscitate Order: Associations With Advance Directives, Physician Specialty and Documentation of Discussion 15 Years After the Patient Self-Determination Act. http://jme.bmj.com/cgi/content/abstract/34/9/642

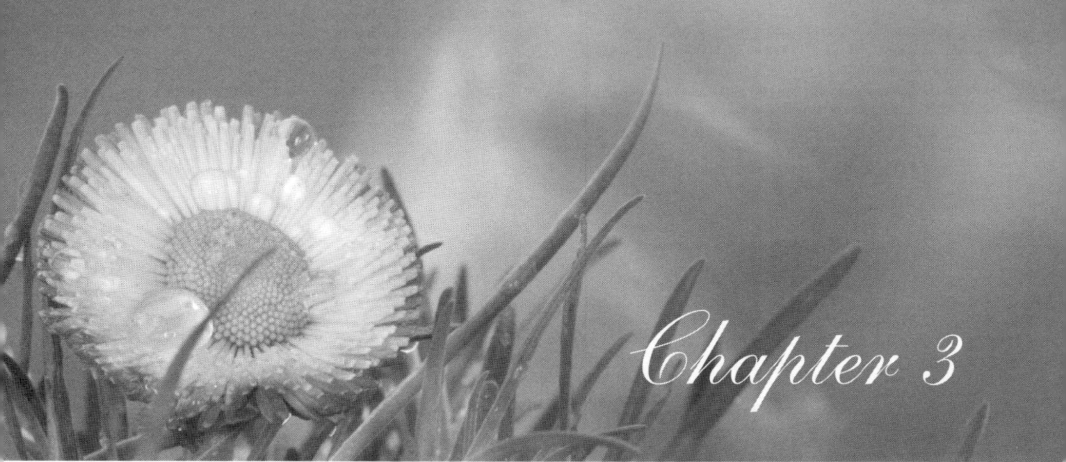

Pain Management

It's More Than Knowing the Meds

I'm not afraid of dying, but I am afraid of pain.

—George, an elderly cancer patient

Listening to the Patient's Pain

Jackie is in her early forties. Two years ago, she was diagnosed with a rare terminal neurological condition. She has gradually lost her ability to control her legs and can no longer walk. As her disease progresses, she is experiencing more pain. During clinic visits and hospitalizations, she has found that both the doctors and the nurses have been reluctant to address her pain.

"They say to me, 'Oh, you can't be in that much pain,' or, 'We don't want to prescribe too much medication because you might become addicted,' or, 'You just have to live with it. That's part of the disease.'"

She is currently hospitalized with a possible bowel obstruction related to the progression of her disease. During this hospitalization her nurse listens to her story and says, "I believe you are in pain. Let's work with the doctor to make you more comfortable."

Jackie begins to cry. "You mean you'll help me?"

Unfortunately, Jackie's story is not unique. Pain is one of the most undertreated conditions in modern medicine. One of the largest scientific studies conducted on care of the dying found that 40 percent of patients who died in the study were in mild to severe pain at the time of their death (Lynn et al., 1997). For those who are dying, pain represents one of the greatest fears. A 1997 Gallup poll asked, "What worries you when you think about your own death?" Sixty-seven percent responded that they were worried about great physical pain before dying (Gallup, 1997).

The role of the nurse in pain management cannot be overemphasized. As skilled clinicians, we need to be competent in assessing pain and understanding the principles of pain management. As advocates, we need to work with physicians and other health care team members to develop the most effective care plan for the patient. As guides, we need to work with the patient and the family to find the highest level of comfort.

The first step is to understand what pain is. Pain can be defined as "an unpleasant sensory and emotional experience associated with actual or potential tissue damage or described in terms of such damage" (Agency for Health Care Policy and Research, 1994, p. 12). More importantly, though, pain is unique to each person and must be defined as *what the patient says it is, existing whenever he or she says it does* (Institute for Clinical Systems Improvement, 2008). As skilled clinicians and advocates, we should not make a subjective judgment on a patient's pain. Remember Jackie's experience: "No one would believe me when I said I had pain." (See the sidebar "Phrases to Avoid.")

Phrases to Avoid

- He doesn't look like he's in pain.
- She couldn't be in pain. It hasn't been 4 hours since her last medication.
- His pain couldn't be *that* bad. The patient in the next bed has a much more serious condition, and he isn't complaining.

Skilled Clinician: Assessment and Management of Pain

Many hospitals, long-term care facilities, and home care agencies are looking at pain as a crucial part of the ongoing patient assessment. Most of us are very familiar with the four major vital signs: temperature, pulse, respirations, and blood pressure. Pain has been added as the *fifth vital sign* and is being assessed on the same schedule.

The first step required in managing pain is to complete a thorough and organized pain assessment. Failure to do so is a common reason for under treatment of pain. (See the sidebar "ABCs of Pain Assessment.")

ABCs of Pain Assessment

Known as the ABCDEF of pain assessment and management, the following is a helpful way of looking at how you can approach a patient.

- A **Ask** about pain regularly. **Assess** pain systematically.
- B **Believe** the patient and family in their reports of pain and what relieves it.
- C **Choose** pain control options appropriate for the patient, family, and setting.
- D **Deliver** interventions in a timely, logical, coordinated fashion.
- E **Empower** patients and their families. **Enable** patients to control their course to the greatest extent possible.
- F **Fine-tune** the pain plan as often as needed.

(Agency for Health Care Policy and Research, 1994; Zerwekh, 2006)

A complete assessment of pain includes the following:

- **Pain history:** When did the pain begin? What is the current medication regimen?
- **Description:** A patient's description of the kind of the pain can help you better assess the most appropriate medication. Words can include dull, aching, gnawing, cramping, shooting, piercing, sharp, or burning.

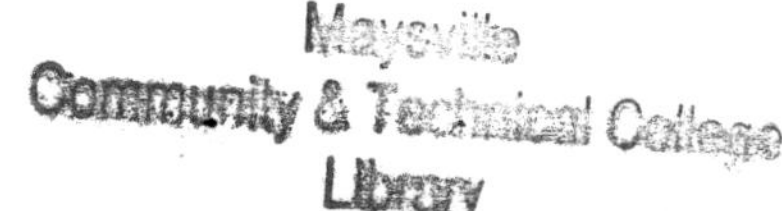

- **Pain intensity or severity rating:** Most pain intensity ratings are variations of a well validated numerical scale of zero to ten, with zero representing no pain and ten indicating the most severe pain imaginable (Daut, Cleeland, & Flanery, 1983). Have patients rate their pain using a pain intensity scale that they can most easily understand. Patients should also be encouraged to keep a log of pain intensity scores at home to report during follow-up visits or phone calls.
- **Location:** Ask the patient to indicate exactly where the pain is occurring and if it radiates. Be aware that it is common for patients to have more than one location and type of pain at any given time.
- **Effects on quality of life:** How does the pain affect the patient? Has it impacted relationships? Does it interrupt sleep? Affect appetite? Increase patient's reliance on others for activities of daily living?
- **Precipitating factors:** What makes the pain worse? Is it associated with certain activities?
- **Relieving factors:** What helps? Is the pain better at certain times? Be aware that patients and families frequently use home remedies in addition to prescribed pain medications. They are also becoming increasingly knowledgeable about complementary therapies, such as acupuncture and homeopathic preparations, but might be hesitant to share these practices with you. Ask specifically if they have tried any complementary therapies and how they have helped.
- **Patient goals:** What is the patient's acceptable level of pain on a zero to ten scale?

A nursing assessment is not complete until you've discussed with the patient and the family the goals of pain control. Do not assume that you know what the patient hopes to achieve—*ask*! Some patients want to be completely pain free, even if it means that they are going to be more sedated. Others are willing to put up with a certain level of pain to be mentally clear. As one patient said, "The morphine makes me pretty sleepy. I want to take a little less today so I can be alert when my 5-year-old granddaughter comes to the hospital to visit."

Some patients, because of age, language and cultural barriers, or cognitive impairment, may be less communicative about their pain. You still need to do as thorough an assessment as possible. This may mean assessing nonverbal signs of pain such as guarding, restlessness, anxiety, combativeness, or facial expressions such as grimacing. Simpler pain assessment tools, picture scales rather than numeric scales, or translated pain assessment tools can be used (Herr et al., 2006). (Note: If you are using the picture scales, understand that these are for patient use, not for matching a patient expression to the picture.)

Principles of Clinical Pain Management

The following principles are based on the classic recommendations of the World Health Organization (WHO, 1990):

- Individualize the treatment regimen to the needs of the patient and family caregivers.
- Use the simplest dosage schedule and least invasive pain management modalities first.
- Follow the WHO three-step analgesic ladder:

  Step One: For mild to moderate pain, use a non-opioid, such as ibuprofen or acetaminophen. Consider adjuvant medications.

  Step Two: For persistent or increasing pain, add an opioid. Consider adjuvant medications.

  Step Three: For continuing pain, or for moderate to severe pain, increase the opioid potency or dose. Consider adjuvant medications. Medicate on a regular schedule, not a p.r.n. (as needed) basis, to ensure consistency in the blood level of the medication. This prevents recurrences of pain. In addition to the regularly scheduled medications, have "breakthrough" or "rescue" doses of pain medication available as needed. *Remember*: As the regularly scheduled dose is increased, the breakthrough dose must also be increased.
- Avoid polypharmacy. The patient should be on only one long-acting opioid for constant pain. The breakthrough drug should be the immediate-release preparation of the sustained-release drug if possible; that is, a patient taking sustained-release morphine should use liquid morphine for breakthrough rather than hydrocodone or hydromorphone.

Important note: One of the most distressing side effects of opioid pain therapy is constipation. The vast majority of patients taking opioids need to be placed on a regularly scheduled bowel program including laxatives and stool softeners. This is essential in ensuring your patient's comfort and avoiding the complications from constipation. Assess and monitor bowel status regularly.

Use of Adjuvant Medications

Adjuvant pain medications enhance the effectiveness of other conventional analgesics and also provide independent analgesia for specific types of pain. You need to understand the role of adjuvant medications as a part of the patient's complete pain regimen. Listed below are common adjuvants and their uses:

- **Tricyclic antidepressants**, as well as newer agents such as duoxetine are effective for neuropathic pain.
- **Anticonvulsants** can be used to manage neuropathic pain, especially pain described as "lancinating" or "burning," or other neuropathic pain that does not respond to antidepressants.
- **Corticosteroids** are useful for severe metastatic bone pain and in reducing pain and headaches associated with cerebral and spinal cord edema.
- **Nonsteroidal anti-inflammatory drugs (NSAIDS)** are the first line treatment for bone metastases and other inflammatory conditions.
- **Topical therapies** such as lidoderm patches have been shown to relieve neuropathic pain.

  Note: Risks should be considered when using these medications. For example, NSAIDs can cause gastrointestinal bleeding and long-term aggressive steriod use can lead to a multitude of complications.

Complementary or Integrative Therapies

A growing body of research is identifying the therapeutic value of nonpharmacy interventions in pain (Lafferty, Downey, McCarty, Standish, & Patrick, 2003; Pan, Morrison, Ness, Fugh-Berman, & Leipzig, 2000; Agency for Health Care Policy and Research, 1994). Complementary or integrative therapies are becoming widely accepted by both the lay public and health care professionals. When nondrug therapies *supplement* the prescribed medication regimen, patients can derive benefit and comfort. In addition, teaching family caregivers complementary therapies that they can easily do to improve the patient's comfort might improve their feelings of being useful and involved in their loved one's care.

Some common complementary approaches to pain management are listed below. Nurses can easily do some of these therapies; others require referrals to the appropriate therapist.

- Massage therapy
- Therapeutic touch
- Physical therapy: exercise, range of motion, ultrasound
- Heat/cold application
- Acupuncture/acupressure
- Relaxation and imagery/meditation

Advocating: Ensuring That the Patient's Pain Relief Goals Are Met

When Helen's mother was admitted to a long-term care facility with terminal breast cancer, she came under the care of a new physician who did not know her well. Helen could see her mother was in pain. "I was fortunate because the charge nurse was so helpful. First, she figured out that Mom needed to be on pain pills on a regular basis. When that still didn't make her comfortable, she was on the phone right away to the doctor to get stronger medication. When the doctor was reluctant to prescribe morphine, the nurse just kept at him and kept at him until we got what we needed for Mom."

The first rule in advocating for your patient is that pain beyond the patient's expressed goal is *unacceptable*. Achieving the acceptable level of comfort might require clinical skills, persistence, and finesse. Start with a thorough patient pain assessment. Perhaps the solution is as simple as working with the physician to change the pain regime from p.r.n. to regularly scheduled doses.

Communication with the physician is essential to advocating for your patient. Be aware that not all physicians are skilled in pain management. However, most care deeply about the needs of their patients. If the physician is struggling with the pain management plan, look for assistance from other team resources. Can the pharmacist help? Does your hospital, long-term care facility, or clinic have access to pain specialists or a palliative care team? Is a hospice program available for a pain consultation?

Communication with the patient and family is another key to advocating for the best pain management. Patients can also pose problems that interfere with good pain relief. For example, many patients are afraid to take opioids because they fear addiction or constipation. Furthermore, many fear that if they start taking a medication like morphine now, they won't be able to have enough pain relief later. Families often have the same concerns. As a son said, "But Dad, I don't want you to become addicted." It is your role to inform, educate, and—above all—to reassure.

The advocacy role does not stop with an initial pain management plan that meets the patient's goals. You need to ask the question, "Is this plan sustainable?" For example, perhaps you have an elderly patient who is on around-the-clock every-4-hour doses of oxycodone while hospitalized. Is it reasonable for the patient to maintain that schedule once he or she is home?

Factors to consider include the following:

- **Future setting for the patient:** Can this plan be maintained at home? In a long-term care facility? Assisted living? Relative's home? This is an excellent time to consult with other team members such as the social worker.
- **Cost:** Medications can be expensive, and they are not always covered by insurance. Is the route, dose, and brand of medicine the most cost-effective? Is the patient eligible for hospice under Medicare? Currently, the Hospice Medicare Benefit covers the cost of pain medication.
- **Cultural considerations:** Make sure the pain management plan is culturally acceptable to the patient and family. In some cultures, the primary decision-maker might be someone other than the patient. If this is the case, the decision-maker must be part of the pain management planning.
- **Potential for abuse:** Misuse and abuse of prescription medications is a significant issue. Be aware that family members, especially teenagers, can be capable of misuse. Can the medication be safely stored or locked up if this is a concern? Some opioids have a "street value" for illegal sale. Does the patient live in a high-risk area? If so, patient safety must be a consideration. Consult with the pharmacist on the best way to manage the medication in these circumstances. Also consider that in high-risk areas, local drug stores might not carry the medication.

As an advocate for the best pain management for your patients, look at the system or organization you work in. Do barriers exist that inhibit timely pain relief for your patients? Does your hospital, long-term care facility, or home care assess pain on a regular basis? If not, what can you do to change the policies? How quickly does your system respond to pain management problems? For example, one hospital discovered that it took nearly 2 hours from the time orders were received on pain management until medication was administered (Lynn, Schuster, & Kabcenell, 2000). By implementing assessment and response standards, the hospital was able to reduce this to 30 minutes.

Guiding Patients and Families: Addressing Common Fears

One of the most important roles you have as a nurse in working with dying patients is that of a guide. This is particularly true in pain management. By understanding the fears that accompany pain, you can guide and teach patients and families.

Fear: Narcotic Addiction

If I take narcotics, I risk becoming addicted.

One of the greatest fears expressed by patients and families about opioids is that taking the narcotics will cause addiction.

Fact

Addiction is defined as a psychological dependence, often resulting in antisocial and destructive behaviors. The literature shows that abuse of therapeutic opioids by patients is rare (Paice & Fine, 2005; Portnoy & Payne, 1992). When you are working with a terminally ill patient, the concern over addiction is irrelevant and harmful in that it interferes with appropriate attention to the comfort and quality of life for the patient.

Fear: Diminishing Returns

If the pain is worse, then my disease is worse. If I take more medication, it will eventually stop working.

Many patients actually underreport their pain for fear that more pain means the disease is getting worse. Others fear that if they take more medication, it will eventually stop working for them.

Fact

Patients with many chronic conditions live well for years on varying doses of opioids and other pain medications. While increased pain can be a sign that the disease is worsening, it does not foreshadow the end of life. Developing tolerance to opioids is generally slow, and all pure opioids (that is, not in combination with other non-opioids such as acetaminophen) have no maximum daily dose or "ceiling" on analgesic effect. In other words, pure opioids can be dosed as high as clinically necessary to achieve pain management.

As a guide, listen to your patients' fears and help them weigh the benefits versus the burdens of their pain management plan. Actively engage both the patient and the family in the pain management plan. (See the sidebar "Engaging the Patient and Family in the Pain Management Plan.")

Engaging the Patient and Family in the Pain Management Plan

You can involve the patient and family by:

- Assessing pain on a regular basis and including the question, "What works best for you?"
- Assuring the patient and family that pain is not an inevitable part of dying.
- Allowing the patient and family to be part of the pain therapy by teaching them about the use of "breakthrough" doses and use of complementary therapies.

Know the Resources

One of the best ways you can be effective in managing your patient's pain is to know the resources. Many excellent books and Web resources provide guidelines on types of pain medications, dosages, and use. If you do not have them available to you at your place of work, ask to have them added to the library or resource shelf. See "Other Resources" at the end of this chapter for some suggestions.

Summary

As a skilled clinician, your first step in managing pain is a thorough assessment. Begin by asking the patient. Know the basics of pain management and use other team resources.

As an advocate, be persistent in ensuring that your patient's pain is managed. Assess your workplace and work to remove barriers to timely and effective pain management. Consider pain as a fifth vital sign.

As a guide, listen to patient and family fears about pain and pain management. Work with the patient and family to dispel myths about pain. Teach the patient and family how to manage pain using both medications and other therapies.

References

Agency for Health Care Policy and Research. (1994). *Management of cancer pain, clinical practice guideline number 6*. Rockville, MD: U.S. Department of Health and Human Services.

Daut, R.L., Cleeland, C.S., & Flanery, R.C. (1983). Development of the Wisconsin brief pain questionnaire to assess pain in cancer and other diseases. Pain 17: pp. 197-210.

George Gallup International Institute. (October 1997). Spiritual beliefs and the dying process: Key findings from a national survey. Nathan Cummings Foundation and Fetzer Institute.

Herr, K., Coyne, P., McCaffrey, M., Manworren, R., Merkel, S., Key, T., Pelosi-Kelly, J., & Wild, L. (2005). Pain assessment in the non-verbal patient: Position statement with clinical practice recommendations. *Pain Management Nursing*. Vol 7. No. 2. pp. 44-52.

Institute for Clinical Systems Improvement. (May, 2008). Health care guideline: Palliative care. Retrieved 14 October 2008 from http://www.icsi.org/palliative_care/palliative_care_11918.html

Lafferty, W., Downey, L. McCarty, R. Standish, L., & Patrick D. (2003). Evaluation CAM treatment at the end of life: A review of clinical trials for massage and meditation. *Complementary Therapies in Medicine.* 14 (2) 100-112.

Lynn, J., et al. (1997). Perceptions by family members of the dying experience of older and seriously ill patients. *Annals of Int. Med.* 126: 97–106.

Lynn, J., Schuster, J.L., & Kabcenell, A. (2000). *Improving care for the end of life: A sourcebook for health care managers and clinicians.* New York: Oxford University Press, p. 41.

Paice, J.A., & Fine, P.G. (2005). *Pain at the end of life.* In Ferrell, B.R., & Coyle, N. (Eds.). *Textbook of palliative nursing (2nd ed.).* New York: Oxford University Press.

Pan, C.X., Morrison, R.S., Ness, J., Fugh-Berman, A., & Leipzig, R.M. (2000). Complementary and alternative medicine in the management of pain, dyspnea, and nausea and vomiting near the end of life: A systematic review. *Journal of Pain and Symptom Management* 20(5): 374–387.

Portney, R.K., & Payne, R. (1992). Acute and chronic pain. In Lowenison, J.H., Ruiz, P., & Millman, R.B. (Eds.). *Substance abuse: A comprehensive textbook (2nd ed.).* Baltimore, Maryland: Lippincott, Williams & Wilkins.

World Health Organization (WHO). (1990). Cancer pain relief and palliative care. Report of a WHO expert committee. Geneva, Switzerland: WHO, pp. 1–75.

Other Resources

Books

Ferrell, B.R., & Coyle, N. (eds.). (2005). *Textbook of palliative nursing, second edition.* New York: Oxford University Press.

Kaye, P. (2006). *Notes on symptom control in hospice and palliative care, revised 2006 edition.* Essex, CT: Hospice Education Institute.

Web resources

City of Hope, Beckman Research Center. http://prc.coh.org/pain_assessment.asp. Comprehensive list of pain assessment guidelines and tools with links.

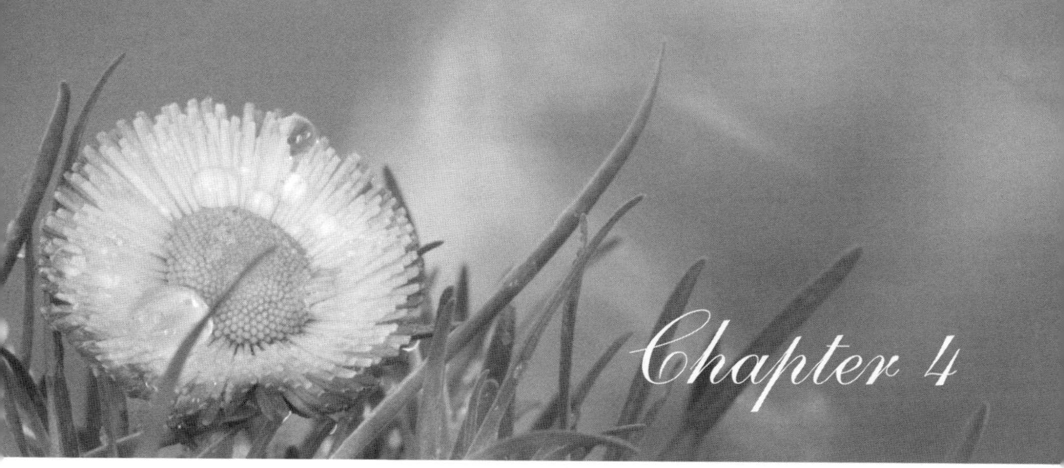

Physical Symptom Management

Knowing What to Look For

Sometimes he would close his eyes and try to draw the air up into his mouth and nostrils, and it seemed as if he were trying to lift an anchor.

—Mitch Albom, *Tuesdays With Morrie*

Common Symptoms

Edgar is a 68-year-old man with end-stage chronic heart failure. He has been hospitalized 3 times in the last 6 months for a variety of problems. He has just been transferred to a skilled nursing facility following a hospitalization for pneumonia. The transfer document indicates a very poor prognosis. When the admitting nurse sees him, he appears to be restless and uncomfortable. However, when she asks him to rate his pain, he says he has none. The nurse then says, "You seem to be so uncomfortable. Can you tell me about it?"

Edgar tells her that sometimes he feels like he can't catch his breath. "I'm afraid I'm going to suffocate, and you won't know what to do."

The nurse says, "Let's see about having some medication on hand in case you feel like you're having trouble breathing." She talks with the doctor and arranges for oxygen and liquid morphine to control his dyspnea.

When patients are dying, they might have many distressing physical symptoms that need to be assessed and addressed. Management of pain is often the primary focus at this time, but a wide array of other problems can cause patients great discomfort (See the sidebar "Common Symptoms Associated with Patients at the End of Life.")

Common Symptoms Associated with Patients at the End of Life

- Dyspnea
- Constipation
- Diarrhea
- Nausea
- Weight loss and loss of appetite (from anorexia and cachexia)
- Skin disorders
- Asthenia and fatigue
- Anxiety
- Depression

Skilled Clinician: Assessment and Management of Common Symptoms

The first step you can take to alleviate the patient's discomfort from these symptoms is a thorough assessment. The assessment includes a medical history and a history of any current symptoms. Questions to ask include the following:

- "Tell me about your health. What is the history of your illness?"
- "Tell me about your most distressing symptoms."

- "Are you having any problems with nausea, constipation, breathlessness, poor appetite, or anything else like that?"
- "What helps these symptoms? What doesn't help?"

A complete symptom assessment also looks into functional status and how symptoms have affected the patient's activities of daily living and relationships. Remember from Chapter 1 that a patient at the end of life wants to be affirmed as a "whole" person. Assessment questions you should ask include the following:

- "Has/have your symptom(s) affected your ability to be independent?"
- "Has/have your symptom(s) affected your family or loved ones?"
- "Have you experienced changes in your routines because of your symptom(s)?"

These questions help you focus on what's truly causing the discomfort for the patient. For example, a patient who is having difficulty with urinary frequency may be less concerned about the physical problem than about the burden on his wife, particularly at night. The nurse can then establish a plan in the hospital that includes reducing fluids in the evening and arranging for a bedside commode to be sent home with the patient at discharge.

In approaching and assessing symptoms, keep in mind that you are looking for the *patient's* perception of the problem above all else. Families sometimes report symptoms or ask for symptom relief for problems that are more distressing to them than they are to the patient. If a family member says, "Do something. He looks so miserable," you need to make sure to ask the patient, "Is this a problem for you?"

Clinical approaches to some of the common symptoms can involve pharmacology as well as basic comfort techniques and complementary therapies.

Dyspnea

Dyspnea, like pain, is a subjective experience and can be one of the most distressing symptoms for patients and their families (Dudgeon, 2005). First, look at the cause. For example, treatment for dyspnea associated with chronic heart failure might include diuretics to relieve fluid build up, whereas treatment for dyspnea associated with anxiety might include antianxiety medications. Common palliative approaches to dyspnea include the following:

- **Oxygen and humidified oxygen via nasal prongs:** Nasal prongs can be irritating to the skin and nostrils. Monitor the skin regularly for signs of irritation.
- **Opioids:** Opioids can be an effective treatment for dyspnea. It is believed that they work by altering the central perception of dyspnea much in the same way they alter the central perception of pain (Dudgeon, 2005).
- **Inhalers and nebulizers:** Saline nebulizers or inhalers with beclomethasone or albuterol used on a regular basis can provide relief. Nebulized morphine can also be an effective and relatively noninvasive way to relieve dyspnea.
- **Anxiolytics:** Breathlessness can be exacerbated by anxiety. A distressing cycle can occur if a patient feels panic because of the dyspnea. Anxiolytics can be used in conjunction with other therapies to relieve the symptoms.

Dyspnea relief can also be achieved without the use of pharmaceutical intervention. (See the sidebar “Simple Remedies to Relieve Breathlessness.”) In addition, you can use complementary therapies. Acupuncture, acupressure, and progressive relaxation have shown some efficacy in relieving breathlessness (Pan et al., 2000).

Simple Remedies to Relieve Breathlessness

- Use a fan to help circulate the air
- Open a window
- Restrict the number of people in the room
- Reposition the patient by elevating the head of the bed

Constipation

The incidence of constipation, especially in cancer patients can be extremely high due to a variety of factors, including use of opioids for pain relief, decreased mobility, and decreased appetite (Economou, 2005). The foremost clinical goal in addressing constipation should be that of prevention. This means you need to routinely assess bowel status, particularly for those patients receiving any type of opioid treatment. Also, when assessing for constipation, ask the patient, "What are your common bowel habits?" You can then adjust therapy to fit the patient's needs. (See the sidebar "Common Treatments for Constipation.")

Common Treatments for Constipation

- **Stimulant laxatives:** These work by stimulating bowel activity. Common ones include senna, casanthranol, and bisacodyl.
- **Osmotic laxatives:** This type of laxative draws water into the bowel. These laxatives include lactulose, milk of magnesia, Miralax, and magnesium citrate.
- **Stool softeners:** These increase the water content of the stool. They include sodium docusate and calcium docusate. A combination of laxative and stool softener is often the most effective for patients taking opioids.
- **Lubricant stimulants and enemas:** Therapies in this category include glycerin suppositories. (Emanuel, von Gunten, & Ferris, 1999)

Dietary and other interventions can also be effective for some types of constipation. Prune juice, for example, works as a stimulant laxative. In putting together a bowel program, ask the patient, "What works best for you?" When asked, one patient said, "Every morning I retire to the bathroom with the crossword puzzle. It's worked for me for years. But here, I can't do that anymore."

Diarrhea

While diarrhea is a less common symptom for patients in the terminal stages of illness, it can be both disruptive and dehumanizing (Muir et al., 1999). It can be caused by a variety of underlying conditions including bowel obstruction, medications, gastrointestinal bleeding, and poor absorption. Common treatments include use of antidiarrheal medications and, in some cases, fluid replacement. You should also consider dietary interventions, such as avoidance of gas-producing foods and lactose.

Nausea and Vomiting

Close to 60 percent of terminally ill patients experience some type of nausea, and 30 percent experience vomiting (Muir et al., 1999). Nausea and vomiting in patients can be caused by a variety of problems ranging from increased cerebral pressure to mechanical obstruction, medications, or infections. The first step in addressing nausea and vomiting is a thorough assessment that includes determining if a pattern exists (i.e., after certain medications, meals, or movement.) (King, 2005). Clinical treatment for nausea and vomiting varies depending on the underlying cause.

Weight Loss and Loss of Appetite

Perhaps one of the most disturbing symptoms for a family to see is the weight loss and loss of appetite in a loved one. We associate nourishment closely with love. When assessing this symptom, find out how the patient feels. Often the patient is far less disturbed by the inability to eat or by the weight loss than the family is. Pharmacologic interventions can include megestrol, prednisone, or dexamethasone to stimulate the appetite and control other symptoms such as nausea and vomiting (Storey, 1996). Nonpharmacologic interventions include the following:

- Offering the patient's favorite foods and nutritional supplements.
- Reducing portion sizes and eliminating dietary restrictions.
- Discussing with the patient and family the natural progression of the disease and what alternatives can be used in place of food to show love and nurturing.
- Using alcohol such as a glass of wine as an appetite stimulant. (First assess for a history of alcohol-related chemical dependency.)

Skin Disorders

The skin is the largest organ in the human body. Because of disease pathology, nutrition, hydration, and mobility issues, terminally ill patients are particularly vulnerable to skin problems. Prevention of skin disorders such as pressure ulcers is the first line of defense. However, sometimes even the most meticulous care cannot stop skin breakdown or discomfort.

Common types of skin problems include the following:

- **Pressure ulcers:** Palliative goals should focus on prevention of further breakdown and management of discomfort and odor (Bates-Jensen, Early, & Seaman, 2001). Pay particular attention to the heels, sacrum, and elbows. Interventions include frequent turning and repositioning, as well as use of specialized pressure-reducing surfaces such as mattress overlays or low-air-loss beds. Meticulous hygiene and positioning are also essential.
- **Pruritus and skin irritation:** Skin itching and discomfort can be a source of great distress for patients. First, start with a thorough assessment including location and description of the discomfort—itching, burning, tickling, "pins and needles." Depending on the type of discomfort, interventions might include thorough cleansing, warm baths, cold packs, and topical creams. Sometimes you might need to use systemic pharmaceuticals such as corticosteroids, antidepressants, or antihistamines to provide relief (Rhiner & Slatkin, 2005).

Fatigue

Loss of energy and tiredness are normal in the progression of a terminal condition, but this fact does not make these conditions any less distressing for the patient or the family. Often helping the patient and family to understand the progression of the disease and to adapt to the patient's fluctuating energy levels can be effective. Patients can also suffer from boredom and understimulation because of inactivity. Encouraging the patient's favorite activities even in a modified form can be restorative (Dean & Anderson, 2005). You can also enlist assistance from other health care team members such as the physical therapist or occupational therapist to suggest ways of helping the patient conserve energy. Pharmacological interventions include the use of steroids or low-dose stimulants.

Anxiety

Many issues can trigger anxiety in a patient facing the end of life. Fear of the future, worry about loved ones, fear of pain, and a general feeling of being overwhelmed by all that is happening can cause distress. Anxiety can be seen in various ways in patients, including increased agitation and restlessness, breathlessness, hyperventilation, and profuse sweating. Pharmacologic treatments include use of medications such as benzodiazapines. Careful assessment and your use of the interdisciplinary team can be keys to relieving anxiety. (See Chapter 5 on suffering.)

Depression

About 50 percent of terminally ill patients experience some type of depression (Muir et al., 1999). By recognizing and managing depression, you can make it possible for the patient and family to not only experience personal growth together but also complete life closure (Emanuel, von Gunten, & Ferris, 1999). Depression can be characterized by persistent feelings of hopelessness and helplessness. Depressed patients express feelings of despair and worthlessness such as, "What good am I to anyone anymore?" Depression is also linked to a vicious cycle with pain for the patient—the more pain patients have, the more depressed they become, and the more depressed they become, the more pain they have. (See the sidebar "Questions to Ask Patients about Depression.")

Questions to Ask Patients about Depression

(Adapted from the PHQ9 Depression Assessment, The MacArthur Initiative)

In the past 2 weeks, how often have you been bothered by the following problems?

- Feeling down, depressed, or hopeless
- Having little interest or pleasure in doing things
- Feeling bad about yourself
- Having thoughts of hurting yourself in some way

The first step in treating depression is to address the distressing physical symptoms such as pain. The second step is to engage other team members including the physician, social worker, or psychologist to create a comprehensive treatment plan. Depression in terminally ill patients can be treated with antidepressant medications, counseling, and alternative therapies such as relaxation and guided imagery. Assess and intervene as early as possible. Patients often don't have the time left that it takes for some interventions, particularly pharmacological-based therapies, to take effect.

In cases of a very short prognosis, low-dose amphetamines can be helpful in lifting the mood. Remember also, not all terminally ill patients are depressed. It's important to distinguish between depression and normal life-closure behavior. For example, a patient can express concern about being a burden to the family without being depressed (Block, 2000).

Advocating: Linking the Needs of the Patient and Family to the Health Care System

As an advocate, you are the link between the needs of the patient and family and the health care system. You need to make sure that the patient receives a comprehensive symptom assessment and that the identified needs of your patient and family are addressed. This means not only charting the assessment but also following through to achieve a comprehensive care plan. The best written assessment is of no use if it's filed away at the back of the chart. For your patient, this might mean the following:

- Immediate discussion with the patient's physician regarding assessed needs.
- Recommendations for other disciplines—social worker, chaplain, dietician, or therapist—to be involved.
- "Watchdogging" orders through the system. It is not acceptable for a patient to be in distress for hours because of a bureaucratic system.

Keep the plan of care patient and family centered. For example, if it's important to the patient to have family members at the bedside, can you change restrictive visiting hours to accommodate this? On the other hand, if the patient is in distress because of too much company, intervene on the patient's behalf. Even small things can make a difference during this difficult time. The wife of a dying patient said, "Even though my husband could not eat, it was important to him that I get my meals. The nurse always ordered a tray and brought it for me. We felt like the hospital really cared."

Know and use the resources available to you. Does your health care center have a palliative care nurse specialist or consult service? Do you have access to hospice care? One of the richest and most comprehensive resources available to patients and families at the end of life is hospice care. Hospice care is available to patients in their place of residence, whether that is a home, a long-term care facility, or some other type of facility. Consider asking the physician for a referral to hospice. (See Chapter 10 on hospice care.)

Guiding Patients and Families: Preparing, Listening, and Assuring

Our nursing role as guides for patients and families can ensure comfort and symptom management. As noted in Chapter 1, patients and families want not only comfort but also preparation for the dying experience. As a guide you can:

- **Assure patients that their symptom needs will be addressed**. For example, you can say, "I know that nausea and upset stomach are distressful for you. We are going to try a new medication. If that doesn't work, we have some other therapies. Here's what you can expect when we start the medication ..."
- **Explain therapies in terms patients and families can understand**. Instead of saying, "We're going to start oxygen at 2 liters per nasal cannula," try, "Sometimes a little extra oxygen can help you breathe better. We're going to start some oxygen that will come through this tube directly into your nose. It will make a little whooshing noise. That way, you know it's on. If it makes you uncomfortable, let us know."
- **Prepare patients and families for what might come next**. "You should find with this new medication that you will be sleepy at first, but after you get used to it, that side effect will go away. It usually takes a day or two."
- **Listen carefully to what the patient and family say about symptoms**. If a patient says, "I get this real anxious feeling at night

when the lights are turned off," you might want to offer to leave the lights on, the curtain open, or the door open.

❖ **Engage the patient and family in the care plan**. Teach the family how to turn and position the patient for more comfort. Ask, "What would you like to know? What are your goals?"

In whatever way you can, always give a clear message to the patient and the family that you are not going to abandon them.

Summary

One of the guiding principles of nursing care at the end of life is relief of undesirable symptoms. As a skilled clinician, you can assess and intervene with a variety of physical symptoms. As an advocate, you can make sure that problems are addressed in a timely manner, that the resources of the team are used, and that your system is hospitable to both the patient and family. As a guide, you can begin preparing the patient and family for death and engage them as much as possible in the care giving and decision making.

References

Albom, M. (1997). *Tuesdays with Morrie.* New York: Doubleday.

Bates-Jensen, B.M., Early, L., & Seaman, S. (2001). Skin disorders. In Ferrell, B.R., and Coyle, N. (eds.). *Textbook of palliative nursing.* New York: Oxford University Press.

Block, S.D. (2000). Assessing and managing depression in the terminally ill patient. *Annals of Internal Medicine* 132: 209–218.

Dean, G.E., & Anderson, P.R. (2005). Fatigue. In Ferrell, B.R., & Coyle, N. (eds.). *Textbook of palliative nursing.* New York: Oxford University Press.

Economou, D.C. (2005). Bowel management:constipation, diarrhea, obstruction and ascites. In: In, Ferrell, B.R., & Coyle, N. (eds.). *Textbook of Palliative Nursing.* New York: Oxford University Press.

Emanuel, L.L., von Gunten, C.F., & Ferris, F.D., (eds.). (1999). The Education in Palliative and End-of-life Care (EPEC) Curriculum: The EPEC Project. The Robert Wood Johnson Foundation. Retrieved 14 October 2008 from http://www.epec.net/EPEC/Webpages/ph.cfm

King, C. (2005). Nausea and vomiting. In, Ferrell, B.R., & Coyle, N. (eds.). *Textbook of Palliative Nursing*. New York: Oxford University Press.

The MacArthur Initiative on Depression and Primary Care. (n.d.). Patient Health Questionnaire (PHQ9). Retrieved September 16, 2008 from www.depression-primarycare.org

Muir, J.C., et al. (1999). Symptom control in hospice: state of the art. *The Hospice Journal* 14: 33–61.

Pan, C.X., et al. (2000). Complementary and alternative medicine in the management of pain, dyspnea, and nausea and vomiting near the end of life: A systematic review. *Journal of Pain and Symptom Management* 20(5): 374–387.

Rhiner, M., & Slatkin, N.E. (2005). Pruritus, fever and sweats. In Ferrell, B. R., and Coyle, N. (eds.). *Textbook of palliative nursing*. New York: Oxford University Press.

Storey, P. (1996). *Primer of palliative care*. Gainesville, FL: American Academy of Hospice and Palliative Medicine.

Other Resources

Doyle, D., Hanks, G.W.C., Cherny, N.I., & Calman, K. (2003). *Oxford textbook of palliative medicine, 3rd edition*. USA: Oxford University Press.

Kaye, P. (2006). *Notes on symptom control in hospice and palliative care*. Essex, CT: Hospice Education Institute.

End of Life/Palliative Education Resources Center (EPERC) Educational Materials. Retrieved 26 October 2008 from http://www.eperc.mcw.edu/

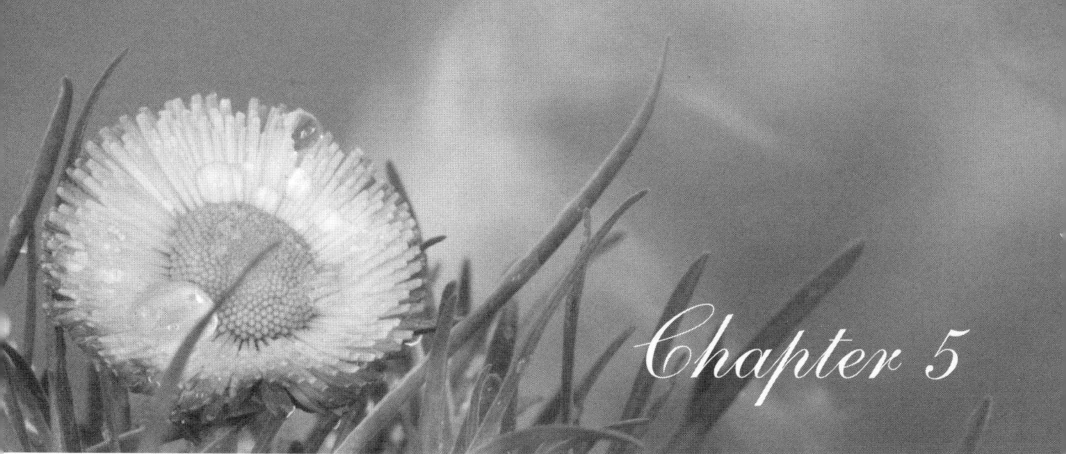

Chapter 5

Suffering

It's Not Just the Pain

Until I did the assessment, neither the patient nor I realized that her distress was not due to her pain, but to her suffering.

—Hospice Nurse

What Is Suffering at the End of Life?

Mrs. S. is an 80-year-old woman with ovarian cancer living alone in her own home. A home-care nurse sees her on a weekly basis. During the visits, the nurse observes that Mrs. S. is restless and unable to sit for long periods of time before she needs to get up and pace. The home-care nurse has asked her on several occasions if she is in pain. Mrs. S. always says, "No." Several medications have been prescribed to help "calm her down." Nothing appears to work. During today's visit, the nurse says, "I'm concerned because you seem so uncomfortable. Is something else going on?"

Mrs. S. starts to cry and says, "I'm afraid to die."

Comfort for a patient doesn't always mean physical symptom relief. To address patients' comfort, you must also address their suffering. In his groundbreaking work on suffering, *The Nature of Suffering*, Dr. Eric Cassel defined suffering as "a state of severe distress associated with events that threaten the intactness of the person" (Cassel, 1991).

The first step in intervening in a patient's suffering is to understand that it is multidimensional and sometimes difficult for a patient to articulate. For nurses who care for dying patients, suffering needs to be looked at in terms of its physical, personal, family, and spiritual aspects.

Skilled Clinician: Assessing Suffering

Your nursing clinical skills in the area of suffering are linked with understanding the concept of suffering, conducting a thorough assessment, and knowing the resources for intervention. Suffering, like pain, should be based on patient report. As with pain, you need to ask and *believe* the patient's response. As noted by Ferrell & Coyle (2008), "Exploring the concept of suffering from the perspective of those who experience it and those who witness it is vital if we are to advance our care." (p. 16.)

Physical Suffering

Not all physical suffering is caused by pain, and not all pain is identified by the patient as physical suffering (Abraham, Kutner, & Beaty, 2006; Baines & Norlander, 2000; Chapman & Gavrin, 1993). Physical suffering can be closely related to issues of quality of life such as independence and self-worth. For example, a patient with amyotrophic lateral sclerosis (ALS) rated his pain very low, but when asked about his physical suffering, rated it very high: "I can no longer raise my hand to my mouth. Do you understand how humiliating it is to not be able to feed yourself anymore?" Another patient rated her physical suffering as very high because she said, "No matter what I try, I'm cold all the time. I hate to get out of bed." Other sources of physical suffering can include the following:

- Physical discomfort that patients don't identify as pain, such as aching, pressure, spasms, cramping, numbness, or tingling.
- Discomfort or distress from immobility. One patient stated, "I can't get out of bed any more and my bones ache."

- Sleeplessness.
- Chills or fever.
- Declining functional ability and increasing dependence on others. As one patient stated, "I used to be able to walk around the block; now I can't walk to the bathroom without resting."
- Changes in appearance, such as weight loss, loss of hair, and disfiguration.
- Skin problems, such as itching, inflammation, or wounds.
- Odors from wounds or diarrhea.

After the source of physical suffering is identified, you can devise a plan of care based on the patient's needs. Your interventions should vary according to the type of distress. (See the sidebar "Key Concepts of Suffering at the End of Life.") For example, if the patient is miserable because of skin itching, you might find medication or regular use of lotions and creams appropriate. If a patient is in distress because of tiredness or weakness, you might consider consulting a physical or occupational therapist to look at ways to conserve patient energy. Or if the patient has identified suffering related to increased dependence on the family for caregiving, you might consider consulting with the social worker to arrange more help for the patient after the patient is discharged to home.

Key Concepts of Suffering at the End of Life

- Suffering is more than pain. It's multidimensional, involving physical, psychosocial, and spiritual aspects.
- Suffering can and should be assessed on a routine basis.
- Not all suffering needs intervention.
- Many interventions for patient suffering are within the nursing skill set.
- Those interventions not within the nursing realm can often be performed by other team professionals.

Personal and Family Suffering

Personal and family distress can have a wide range of implications. Suffering in this area can be related to relationships, unfinished business, grief, or fears of the future. Some patients have difficulty expressing themselves in this area. Questions you should ask include the following:

- **How much are you suffering because of loss of enjoyment of life?** A patient with chronic obstructive pulmonary disease (COPD) said, "Golf was everything to me. Now I can't play anymore, and I sit here day after day just thinking about being outside."
- **How much are you suffering because of your feelings for and relationships with family and friends?** A hospice nurse visited a dying patient at home for the first time. She said, "The patient was in terrible pain. Yet, when I asked her about what she wanted, she told me the most important thing to her was not relieving the pain; it was reconciling with her daughter. The first thing I did was arrange for the daughter to come over with a social worker present."
- **How much are you suffering because of your concern for your loved ones?** A patient who rated his suffering high in this area said, "My wife doesn't even know how to write a check. What's going to happen when I'm gone?"
- **How much are you suffering because of fear of the future?** When asked this question, an elderly patient replied, "I'm afraid those doctors are going to do things to me to try to keep me alive. I don't want to be a vegetable in a long-term care facility."
- **How much are you suffering because of unfinished business?** A young mother told the nurse, "I want to leave something for my daughters to remember me by, but I'm so sick now I can't think what to do for them."

Suffering in the psychosocial realm encompasses a lifetime of beliefs and relationships. With your daily workload, you might not have enough time with patients to adequately address all these issues. However, one of the most important clinical skills you can offer to patients is the ability to listen and acknowledge the distress. As Dr. Ira Byock has noted, "The optimal way to know the experience of another person is to ask" (1996, p. 243). You also have the powerful ability to offer the resources of other professional team members including social workers, therapists, and chaplains.

Spiritual Suffering

Perhaps one of the most difficult areas for you to assess, yet one of the most important for patients at the end of life, concerns the realm of spirituality. Some have also identified this as existential suffering (Cherny, Coyle & Foley, 1994). Others have called it the search for meaning, for hope, or for connections with oneself, others, or a higher power (Corr, C., Nabe & Corr, D., 2000). Spirituality extends beyond issues of religion and faith and into the realm of the meaning of life.

A middle-aged woman expressed the complexity of this concept when she recalled her mother's death when she was 16. "A few weeks before she died, mom looked at me with such anguish in her eyes and asked, 'What was it all about?' She wouldn't live to see me grow up, to see her grandchildren, and to realize some of her own dreams. At 16, I didn't know what to say to her. At 50, I still don't know the answer."

For assessing a patient in this realm, you can ask the following helpful questions:

- **How much are you suffering relative to your ability to interact with your spiritual (or faith or religious) tradition?** An elderly homebound man expressed a high degree of suffering in this area because he had regularly attended church in his community and received communion before being ill. Now that he couldn't get out of the house, he missed his weekly communion.
- **How much are you suffering relative to your ability to find strength in your belief system?** Patients might respond to this question with statements about feeling abandoned by their higher power.
- **How much are you suffering relative to your feelings about your personal source of inner strength?** This question can bring up feelings of hopelessness or inadequacy. For example, a patient might respond, "I used to think I was the strong one in the family, but I'm no good anymore."

Your nursing intervention in the area of spiritual suffering begins with listening and acknowledging the distress. You cannot provide meaning for another, but you can encourage patients to tell their own stories. You can also ask, "Would you like help in this area?" Again, remember you can offer the resources of the other professionals on your health care team.

Advocating for Patients: Ensuring a Holistic View

Because assessing patient suffering at the end of life can be complex and extends well beyond some of the daily tasks of nursing, you can easily fall into the pattern of looking only at physical symptoms and needs. As an advocate for the patient and the family, you are essential in seeing that the patient is viewed holistically. On a patient/family level this means you need to address suffering as a routine part of your comprehensive patient comfort assessment. Just as you ask a patient, "Can you rate your pain on a zero to ten scale?" You can also ask, "Can you rate your physical, personal, family, and spiritual suffering on a zero to ten scale?"

As an advocate, be prepared to look for ways to honor your patient's wishes. Patient suffering can be increased by confinement in an unfamiliar bed in an unfamiliar room. Many patients at the end of life want to spend their final time in the comfort of their own home. Consider what you can do to facilitate a discharge to home:

- Advocate for a hospice or home-care referral.
- Teach the patient and family the necessary care activities before discharge.
- Simplify the medication regime (IV to oral, short-acting opioids to sustained-release opioids).

If care at home is not possible, what can you do to make the hospital or long-term care facility more home-like? The first place to start in accommodating the patient and family is to ask them, "What can we do to make you more comfortable?"

Within your health care institution—hospital, long-term care facility, home-care agency, or clinic—you can also advocate for routine suffering and comfort assessments for patients who are dying. Be prepared, however, to meet some resistance. One of the great fears you might have in addressing patient suffering is that you will ask the question, the patient will answer, and you will not know how to intervene. Remember the following when asking yourself whether you are prepared to address patient suffering:

- Listening and acknowledging patient suffering can be an intervention in itself.
- Not all patients want or need intervention in suffering.

- Many interventions, such as active listening, are already part of your nursing skill set.
- You have other interdisciplinary team members who can help.

Guiding Patients and Families: Start with Yourself

For patients who are suffering at the end of life, your skills as a guide are crucial. As you ask yourself, "What can I do to help guide this patient and this family?" Remember that the first place to start is with yourself. How comfortable are you caring for a dying patient? A new graduate nurse recalled her first experience with a dying patient. "I cared for him as quickly as possible and got out of the room. I could see in his eyes that he was suffering, but I was so afraid he might die while I was with him and I wouldn't know what to do." Your fears and uncertainty can be communicated to the patient and to the family in many ways.

If you are not comfortable caring for someone who is dying, ask yourself why. If you can answer that question, you can grow into your nursing practice. Possible answers include:

- **I've never done this before.** You will face death at some time in your career, either professionally or personally. Read about nursing care for those who are dying. You will find excellent resources available. Attend professional education seminars. Talk with your colleagues.
- **I'm afraid I'll do something wrong.** Remember, you are not alone in caring for the patient. You have other professionals. Use them. And use your listening skills. Patients at the end of life need to tell their story. Families need to be heard.
- **What if the patient has a problem I can't fix?** Not all symptoms, suffering, or distress at the end of life can be "fixed." The message to convey to patients and families is this: "I will not abandon you, and I will do everything in my power to make things more comfortable."

As a guide to the patient and family, you need to be *present* for them. A nurse who efficiently bathes a patient, changes a dressing, or administers a medication is not necessarily *present*. Presence means listening, touching, acknowledging, and honoring a patient's wishes.

Listening

Listening to a dying patient can be both verbal and nonverbal. You can guide the patient who wants to talk by using open-ended questions such as "Can you tell me more?" Or you can use affirming statements such as, "That must be hard for you." Sometimes sitting silently with a patient can be the most effective form of listening.

Acknowledging

Patients who are at the end of life's journey state they want to be acknowledged as still having something to contribute (Steinhauser et al., 2000). Guidance can include encouraging patients to tell or write their life stories and experiences. This can be done on audio or video, through the creation of an ethical will (a nonlegal document that includes items such as values, beliefs, and life's lessons for family, friends, and community) or through letters. For example, with the encouragement and assistance from a nurse, a young woman dying from breast cancer wrote letters to both her young daughters to be opened on their birthdays each year until they were 18.

Touching

Sometimes families are afraid to touch their loved one for fear they might "disconnect" something such as an IV or a monitor. You can guide families through example and by teaching them simple tasks such as turning, positioning, and massage. You can also guide through your own example. Sit when talking with the patient. Provide gentle touch as is comfortable for the patient.

Honoring the Patient's Wishes

Patient wishes near the end of life are varied. Your first step in honoring those wishes is to simply ask, "What would you like?" When asked what he would really like to have, one home-care patient answered, "A lobster tail." With the encouragement of the nurse who assured the family that at this point in the illness a low-fat, low-salt diet was not necessary, the family prepared a lobster dinner. While the patient ate very little of it, he loved the festiveness of the occasion.

Summary

One of the guiding principles of nursing care at the end of life is addressing patient suffering. As the nurse for a dying patient, you are in the most powerful position to intervene with that patient's suffering. Your clinical skills include the ability to assess suffering, intervene where appropriate, and refer to other professional team members. As an advocate, you can work with your institution to make sure that suffering at the end of life is routinely assessed and that barriers to a patient's comfort are removed. As a guide, you can be *present* for the patient and family, acknowledge their suffering, and listen to their needs.

References

Abraham, A., Kutner, J.S., & Beaty, B. (2006). Suffering at the end of life in the setting of low physical symptom distress. *Journal of Palliative Medicine* 9(3): 658–665.

Baines, B., & Norlander, L. (2000). The relationship of pain and suffering in a hospice population. *The American Journal of Hospice and Palliative Care* 17(5): 319–326.

Byock, I.R. (1996). The nature of suffering and the nature of opportunity at the end of life. *Clinics in Geriatric Medicine* 12(2): 237–252.

Cassel, E.J. (1991). *The nature of suffering and the goals of medicine.* New York: Oxford University Press, p. 33.

Chapman, C.R., & Gavrin, J. (1993). Suffering and its relationship to pain. *Journal of Palliative Care* 9: 5–13.

Cherny, N.I., Coyle, N., & Foley, K.M. (1994). Suffering in the advanced cancer patient: a definition and taxonomy. *Journal of Palliative Care* 10(2): 57–70.

Corr, C.A., Nabe, C.M., & Corr, D.M. (2000). *Death and dying, life and living.* Belmont, CA: Wadsworth/Thomson Learning.

Ferrell, B.R., & Coyle, N. (2008). *The nature of suffering and the goals of nursing.* New York: Oxford University Press.

Steinhauser, K., et al. (2000). In search of a good death: Observations of patients, families and providers. *Annals of Internal Medicine* 132(10): 825–832.

Other Resources

Baines, B. (2006). *Ethical wills* (2nd ed.). Cambridge, Massachusetts: De Capo Press.

Ethical Wills: http://www.ethicalwill.com

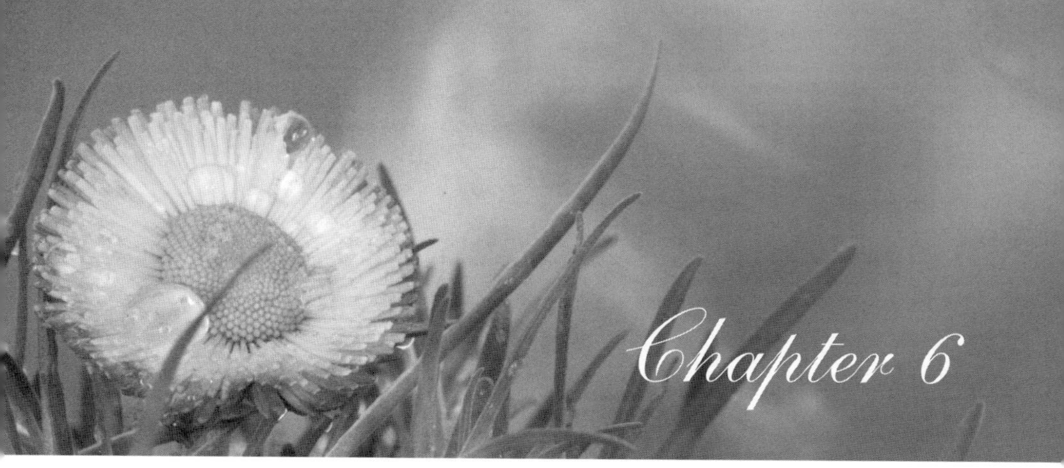

Active Dying

The Final Days and Hours

Wally gave us a gift in the last week of his life: the opportunity to gather as a family, to laugh, to tell stories, and to say good-bye.

—Daughter-in-law of a hospitalized patient

Active Dying: What Does It Mean?

Mrs. N. is an 87-year-old widow who suffered a massive cerebrovascular accident (stroke) 5 days ago. No improvement has been noted after several days of active treatment. Mrs. N.'s family has made the decision to forego further treatment including the placement of a feeding tube. The IV hydration was discontinued 2 days ago. Mrs. N. is no longer responding to verbal stimulation. Her breathing is labored. The family has been keeping a bedside vigil and is becoming more anxious. They ask the nurse caring for Mrs. N., "Is there something more we should be doing? She seems to be struggling to breathe."

The nurse replies, "What you are seeing with her breathing is a normal part of the body slowing down. I'd like to talk with you more about what you can expect to see as she changes."

Nurses who work regularly with dying patients often refer to the final phase of life as the period of active dying. This is the time when physiological and mental changes signal that the patient's bodily functions are shutting down. For the patient and family, this can be a momentous time of completion. You need to include the patient and family in the decision making and care at this time. What happens in those last days and hours can leave a lasting impression on those who live on.

Skilled Clinician: Assessing and Intervening When Death Is Near

To treat some of the symptoms associated with active dying, you must first understand and then assess what is occurring in the dying patient's body. Several clinical indicators can signal that death is close. (See the sidebar, "Clinical Indicators That Death Is Near.")

Clinical Indicators That Death Is Near

- Increased fatigue and weakness
- Decreased food and fluid intake
- Breathing changes
- Skin color changes
- Decreased levels of consciousness
- Other signs: Loss of sphincter control, grimacing and involuntary body jerks, and the inability to close eyes

Increased Fatigue and Weakness

As patients near death, their strength and tolerance for activity decreases. Sometimes this is a gradual process over a period of months or weeks, and sometimes it is quite sudden, with changes happening over a period of days. As patients become weaker and are more likely to be confined to bed, nursing care needs to be focused on both patient and family comfort.

For the bed-bound patient, frequent turning, repositioning, and meticulous skin care are essential. You have the opportunity at this time to engage the family in caregiving by teaching positioning and skin care. Explaining clearly to the family what is happening can help to alleviate their anxiety. Be prepared to explain in simple terms that the weakness is because the body is "giving out," not a sign that the patient is "giving up."

Decreased Food and Fluid Intake

One of the most distressing aspects of a patient's dying for families is seeing a loved one stop eating and drinking. We associate food and fluid with the essence of life, so families at this time express fears such as, "But if he doesn't eat, he'll starve," and "If he's not drinking, won't he feel thirsty?" On the other hand, most patients do not express feelings of either hunger or thirst (Berry & Griffie, 2005; Printz, 1992).

You can help patients and families in the following ways:

- Listen to the family concerns and provide information about decreased food and fluid intake as part of a natural process. If families ask about hydration, you can indicate to them that many studies have shown that it can actually increase patient discomfort in the last days of life (Berry & Griffie, 2005; Emmual, von Gunton, & Ferris, 1999). (See the sidebar "Discomfort with Hydration.")
- Encourage family members to use alternative care. For example, teach the family how to provide mouth care.
- Encourage the family to provide comfort to the patient through touch, music, conversation, or gentle massage.

Discomfort with Hydration

- Intravenous needles and catheters can cause local discomfort.
- Artificial hydration can cause fluid overload and increased swelling in a patient.
- Artificial hydration can contribute to shortness of breath, congestion, and breathing difficulty.

Breathing Changes

The patient who is dying often does not experience distress as breathing patterns change. However, the family can view the changes as indications that the patient is in discomfort. For example, a patient's breathing pattern changing to very rapid is normal, but the family might ask if the patient is feeling air hunger or is suffocating. You might want to prepare families for these common changes as death nears:

- **Periods of very rapid breathing interspersed with periods of very slow breathing:** Use of oxygen does not appear to be of either help or hindrance.
- **Periods of apnea:** Patients might breathe normally, then stop for short periods of time, and then resume normal breathing. Families describe trying to "breathe for the patient" during the periods of apnea.
- **Congestion or gurgling noises:** Sometimes known as the *death rattle,* this phenomenon is perhaps one of the most upsetting aspects of active dying for families. This is the gurgling sound associated with secretions accumulating in the upper part of the patient's respiratory track. Suctioning is not recommended because it often cannot reach the secretions and because it causes distress to the patient. You can treat this effectively with frequent repositioning of the patient and restriction of fluids. You will also find anticholinergic drugs such as scopolamine or atropine that dry secretions to be helpful (Zerwekh, 2006). If a patient is receiving IV hydration and patient respirations are becoming noisy, you might use that as a good time to discuss discontinuing fluids with the family.
- **Agonal breathing:** You can see agonal breathing as a shallow pursing of the lips, like that of a fish out of water. This type of breathing is generally what you see just before a patient dies and can be taken as a signal that death is near.

Skin Color Changes

As the body slows down, so does the circulation of the blood. Skin in the extremities can turn a mottled bluish color. Often you first note this coloring in the feet, hands, and knees. The mottling can progress up the body. Along with color changes, you should notice extremities beginning to cool. This can be particularly distressing to families, who often ask, "Is he or she cold? Should we use more blankets?" You can provide assurances that this is an expected part of this stage of dying and that the patient is in no distress.

Changes in Levels of Consciousness, Confusion, and Delirium

Patients who are close to dying often sleep more deeply and become less and less arousable. They might moan or jerk in their sleep. When awake, they might be very clear or very confused. Sometimes they might say things that make no sense to the family. Patients might talk about doors or windows or even maps. Some, including Maggie Callanan and Patricia Kelley in their book *Final Gifts: Understanding the Special Awareness, Needs, and Communications of the Dying*, call this symbolic language or "nearing death awareness" (Callanan & Kelley, 1992).

Prepare the family for some of these common changes:

- **Confusion:** Patients often arouse confused about time or place. In addition, they sometimes describe seeing people in the room who have died before them such as a parent or spouse. Assure the family that this is normal and acknowledge the patient by saying, "I don't see what you are seeing. Are you comfortable?" Reorient the patient to person, time, and place as necessary.
- **Terminal delirium:** Sometimes a patient who has been quiet, even unresponsive, can have a brief burst of energy. It can take the form of restlessness or agitation. Some have described this as heralding "the difficult road to death" (Emmual, Von Guten, & Ferris, 1999). When this happens, families often mistake this behavior for pain. Increased pain medication generally is not effective. Benzodiazapenes administered orally or buccally have been effective in calming some patients. Again, assure the family and prepare them for this.

Other Signs

You should be watchful for other signs that a patient is nearing death:

- **Loss of sphincter control:** The patient can become incontinent of urine and stool. Pay careful attention to keeping the patient clean and dry.

- **Decreased urine output or inability to urinate:** As the kidneys shut down, urine output decreases. However, do not assume that decreased urine output automatically means kidney failure. As the body slows down, sometimes patients lose the ability to urinate independently. Palpate for a full bladder and observe for signs of agitation or pain. Urinary catheter placement might be necessary.
- **Moaning, grimacing, and involuntary body jerks:** Changes in the central nervous system can lead to these symptoms. Patients can also demonstrate a "picking" behavior where it appears they are picking at objects floating in the air. The best management for these symptoms is to prepare the family and assure them that they do not indicate that the patient is uncomfortable.
- **Inability to close eyes:** Families can be very distressed when they see their loved one with eyes only partially closed and the whites exposed. This symptom happens because of tissue wasting around the eye and eyelid. Use lubricating eye drops as needed to keep the patient comfortable.

Patients die in their own unique ways. Not all signs are going to be present. When you are preparing the family for this final stage, explain in brief and simple terms what they might expect and assure them that you are not going to abandon them.

A Note on Pain

Little evidence exists that pain increases as a patient nears death. Continue to assess and treat for pain. Continue regularly scheduled pain medications. Be careful not to overtreat by mistaking some of the common neurological symptoms such as grimacing or moaning as signs of increased discomfort from pain. However, remember that clinicians tend to undertreat rather than overtreat pain. If you have pain management concerns, consider it a good time to consult with another team member such as the physician, pharmacist, or palliative care nurse to determine the best course.

Advocating for Both the Patient and Family: Communication Is the Key

As the death of the patient nears, you might find yourself in conflicting roles as an advocate for both the patient and the family. These are highly charged emotional times for the family. They often look to you to "do something." In a moment of panic, they might ask for resuscitation, IV fluids, dialysis, or other aggressive measures, even if the patient has clearly stated wishes to the contrary. Your communication skills are key here, along with your use of the other team members. If the patient is actively dying and the family wants a change from comfort to aggressive care, your response should be, "Let's involve the doctor and talk about this as a family." Oftentimes, the family needs reassurance that no "last ditch" measures can keep the patient alive. You might also see this as the time to call in the chaplain or community clergy to talk with the family.

The last phase of dying can be a sacred time for families, a time to tell stories and a time to say good-bye. As an advocate for the patient and family, consider what you can do to facilitate an intimate and comfortable environment. If you are in a hospital or long-term care facility setting, can the patient be transferred to a private room? What can be done to provide more space for the family? Can you arrange for space for the family to bring in favorite photos or mementos? Always consider the importance of respecting cultural beliefs related to the dying process. Ask what you can do to accommodate those needs.

Families often have little experience caring for or being with someone who is dying. Do you have written resources available to them that can help prepare them for what is to come? If not, advocate that your institution or agency add these materials as part of patient education.

Clinically, at this time you need to assess the treatments the patient is receiving. Many treatments and procedures that are routine might no longer be necessary and may actually cause the patient discomfort (Brody, Campbell, Faber-Langendoen, & Ogle, 1997). Look at the following:

- Daily lab tests
- Frequent assessment of vital signs
- Routine weights
- Any procedure that does not promote the comfort of the patient

Guiding: Walking That Difficult Path

The patient and family are looking to you as a guide to walk with them through a very difficult time. To do this, you must be confident and competent in understanding what happens during the final days and hours of life. You must be able to communicate well to the patient and family in terms they can understand. Avoid using highly technical terms such as *terminal delirium*, *dyspnea*, *Cheyne-Stokes breathing*, or *neurological dysfunction*. The phrase *active dying* can also be confusing for the family. (See the sidebar "Phrases to Use.")

Phrases to Use

Phrases might include the following:

- "His breathing is changing. He might stop for a few seconds and then start again. This is normal, and it's not uncomfortable for him."
- "Often patients see people from their past. This does not mean that he is 'out of his head.' We don't know why it happens, but it seems to provide great comfort for the person."
- "It's not unusual to see the blood pressure drop or the heart speed up. This is part of the body slowing down. It is not uncomfortable."

Families often need guidance at the bedside when the patient is near death and sometimes ask the question, "What should we be doing?"

Suggestions you can give them include the following:

- Assign caregiving tasks, such as mouth and skin care, to family members.
- Teach the family how to do simple complementary therapies such as hand massage.
- Offer the services of the chaplain or offer to contact someone from the family's faith community. Patients and families often find comfort in religious ritual as death nears.
- Suggest the use of music. Note, however, that music is a very personal preference. Do not tune into a music station or play music without the input of the patient or the family.

- Encourage the family to tell stories. Remember, even if patients appear to be unresponsive, you do not know what they can hear. Model for the family by talking to the patient rather than talking "over" the patient.
- Encourage the family to perform comfortable family rituals such as singing favorite songs, reading passages from a religious text such as the Bible or Qur'an (also called the Koran) or a favorite book, or reciting familiar prayers.
- Guide the family in saying good-bye. Families sometimes need suggestions of words to use. Consider simple phrases such as "I love you," "I'll miss you," and "Good-bye."

Perhaps the most important role you can play as a guide is to assure the family that there is no right way and no wrong way to do this. Their presence alone is one of the greatest gifts a family can give to a dying patient.

A Note on Withdrawing Life-Sustaining or Life-Extending Treatment

Nurses working in critical care units are sometimes faced with the emotional and clinical complexities surrounding the withdrawal of life-sustaining treatments. This often includes discontinuing mechanical ventilation, dialysis, and artificial nutrition and hydration. During these situations, you must attend to both the comfort of the patient and the needs of the family (Brody, Campell, Faber-Langendoen, & Ogle, 1997). Know the resources available to ensure the best palliation of symptoms during the withdrawal process and use the expertise of other team members including the physician, pharmacist, chaplain, and social worker.

Summary

One of the guiding principles of nursing care at the end of life is to prepare the patient and family for death. As a patient is dying, you need to have strong clinical skills to assess and intervene with some of the symptoms associated with active dying. Your communication skills are important as you need to explain to the patient and family what is happening and what to expect. Your advocacy includes making sure that families have a safe and comfortable place to be with the patient and that unnecessary treatments and procedures are discontinued. Perhaps one of your most important nursing interventions at this time is the guidance you can provide to patients and families concerning communication, rituals, and life "completion."

References

Berry, P., & Griffie, J. (2005). Planning for the actual death. In: Ferrell, B.R., & Coyle, N. (eds.) *Textbook of Palliative Nursing*. New York: Oxford University Press.

Brody, H., Campbell, M.L., Faber-Langendoen, K., & Ogle, K.S. (1997). Withdrawing intensive life-sustaining treatment—recommendations for compassionate clinical management. *The New England Journal of Medicine* 336(9): 652–657.

Callanan, M., & Kelley, P. (1992). *Final gifts: understanding the special awareness, needs, and communications of the dying*. New York: Bantam Books.

Emanuel, L.L., von Gunten, C.F., & Ferris F.D., eds. (1999). The education in palliative and end-of-life care (EPEC) curriculum: The EPEC project. The Robert Wood Johnson Foundation. Retrieved November 3, 2008 from http://www.epec.net/EPEC/Webpages/ph.cfm.

Printz, L.A. (1992). Terminal dehydration, a compassionate treatment. *Archives of Internal Medicine* 152: 697–700.

Zerwekh, J.V. (2006). *Nursing care at the end of life: palliative care for patients and families*. Philadelphia: F.A. Davis, pp. 179–211.

Other Resources

End of Life/Palliative Education Resource Center (EPERC). http://www.eperc.mcw.edu/

Karnes, B. (1995). *Gone from my sight: The dying experience*. Stillwell, Kansas: Barbara Karnes. This is a simply written resource for families on the dying process.

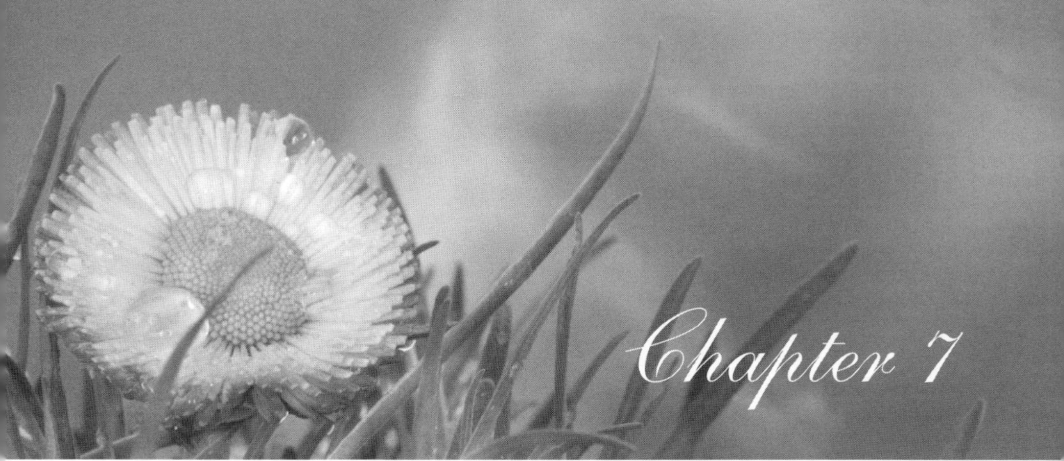

After the Death

The Long Journey to the Car

The longest walk in the world is from the room where you have left your loved one, or watched them leave with the funeral home, to the car that is now taking you to an emptier house.

—The Rev. Chuck Meyer (Meyer, 2000)

What Happens after a Patient Dies?

Mr. F., a 69-year-old married man with a history of heart problems, is admitted to the coronary care unit following a massive heart attack. After several days of treatment, he arrests, and attempts to restart his heart are unsuccessful. His wife and two daughters sit numbly in the waiting room as the doctor explains what happened. Recognizing their state of shock and distress, Mr. F.'s nurse asks, "Would you like to be with your husband for awhile?" She and another nurse quickly clean up the room and remove equipment. She brings the family in, makes sure they are comfortable, and then asks, "Is there anyone you'd like me to call?"

When a death occurs, nurses continue to be responsible for the well-being of both the patient and the family. The well-being of the patient includes respect for the body and the person the body represents. The well-being of the family means respect and understanding of their grief.

Skilled Clinician: Understanding Grief

Grief is an individual manifestation of loss and is influenced by factors ranging from age to previous history with death to coping ability (Zerwekh, 2006). Grief manifests in a variety of ways: emotionally, psychologically, and physically. You might see a variety of reactions in someone who has experienced an immediate loss including sadness, anger, anxiety, confusion, or numbness. Family members might also experience physical reactions such as weakness, dry mouth, or shortness of breath (Worden, 1991).

Your communication skills as a nurse are important to the clinical management of grief following the death of a patient. How you respond to the family can leave a lasting impression on them. If the death was expected and the family was able to be at the bedside, your first intervention should be a sincere and sympathetic acknowledgement of the death. Saying, "*I am sorry for your loss*," is powerful and appropriate.

If the death was unexpected or sudden, you can provide a quiet, comfortable place to talk with the family. It is *inappropriate* to talk with a family about a death in a public waiting room or corridor. Sit down when you talk with the family. Use a preparatory phrase such as, "I'm sorry, the news is not good." Explain in simple, nontechnical terms; stop and let the family talk (Emanuel et al., 1999). (See the sidebar "Nursing Interventions after the Death.")

Nursing Interventions After the Death

- Allow the family time to be with the body.
- Observe the family for signs of distress that warrant intervention.
- Listen actively. Often families need to tell their stories.

Families might feel emotionally numb or simply lost. Ask concrete questions. Rather than saying, "*Can I do anything for you?*" try "*Can I get you a glass of water?*" or "*Would it be all right if I called the chaplain?*"

If you are unable to stay with the family, provide assurance that you are available to them. You might want to set some definite times with them, such as "I'll be back in 15 minutes. If you need me sooner, you can turn on the call light."

If a family member is having a particularly difficult time and manifesting serious physical symptoms such as chest pains or shortness of breath, involve the physician for assessment and treatment. Be aware that other professional team members such as the chaplain or social worker might provide comfort and assistance at this time.

Sometimes immediate grief might manifest itself in the form of anger or accusations: "Why didn't you do more for him?" Acknowledge the anger and listen in a nonjudgmental way.

Families also are going to have questions about what to do next. You might face questions about organ donation, autopsy, and arrangements for the body and for the funeral. Know your institution's policies and procedures regarding after-death care.

As a skilled clinician, you need to recognize that the patients you are caring for might be grieving a loss or have multiple loss issues. Acknowledge those losses and listen with compassion when your patients and families talk about them.

Advocating for the Family: Accommodating Their Comfort Needs

Advocating for the family after the death takes several forms. First and foremost, you can provide a quiet, comfortable place for the family. If you work in a hospital or long-term care facility, find space away from public waiting rooms and corridors. Facilitate private, quiet time for the family to spend with the body. Families should not be rushed during this time. For some, this is the last time they see their loved one, a time to say good-bye.

Respect cultural beliefs and preferences. As much as possible, accommodate the family's needs. This accommodation might range from specific rituals at the bedside to family involvement in washing and clothing the body before it is removed from the room.

Provide professional resources for the family. If they have questions about the medical treatment, arrange for them to spend time with the physician. Facilitate access to chaplains and social workers.

Whether you practice nursing in a hospital, clinic, long-term care facility, or home setting, bereavement follow-up needs to be a part of any patient plan of care. Work within your system to ensure that written resources are available to the family. Some hospitals and institutions have prepared pamphlets that answer some of the immediate questions following a death, such as how to handle organ donation, autopsies, funeral arrangements, and death certificates. Every death needs to be acknowledged in some form. Unfortunately, for many families whose loved one has died in an institution, the only contact they have after the death is with the billing department. (See the sidebar "Suggestions for Your Health Care Institution or Agency.")

Suggestions for Your Health Care Institution or Agency

- Send a sympathy card to the family. Cards should be culturally sensitive, that is, without a strong religious message.
- Provide bereavement follow-up materials, via mail, if necessary, such as information on grief groups.
- Keep a bedside journal where the professional staff can write a note about the patient. This journal can then be sent home with the family.

Guiding the Family: Accepting the Loss

Often your nursing involvement following the death of the patient is short term. However, you still need to understand what the family is going to face as they mourn the loss of a loved one. Normal grieving involves four tasks (Worden, 1991):

1. Accepting the reality of the loss
2. Working through the pain
3. Adjusting to a life without the loved one
4. Moving on with life

As you guide the family through the initial loss, you can be especially helpful in the area of accepting the reality of the loss. Acceptance often begins at the bedside while the patient is dying. Encourage the family to be with the patient. As one daughter said, "We sat around Dad's bed, chatting to each other and to him. Suddenly, as a family we *knew* he was about to leave us. No one said anything, we just *knew*. We stopped talking and held hands and were with him when he slid gently away. I wouldn't give those moments up for anything."

Acceptance of the loss comes easier if the family has the opportunity to see the body and to touch it. Ask the family members if they would like to prepare the body in any way. Some find comfort in providing that last bath. For families who do not want to participate in the preparation, remove equipment, lines, and clutter from the room.

If you are providing nursing care in a hospital, long-term care facility, or other institution, do not forget "the long walk to the car." When the family is ready to leave, offer to accompany them to the car. Your *presence* sends the message that their loved one had meaning to those who provided care before the death.

In guiding families, be sure you avoid the pitfalls of using clichéd and misguided phrases. (See the sidebar "Clichés and Misguided Phrases.")

Clichés and Misguided Phrases

"Be Strong" Clichés

"You must be strong for your children. You have to get hold of yourself. Don't cry."

Instead, say, "*It's OK to cry. I'm so sorry. Would you mind if I sat with you for a few minutes?*"

Religious Clichés

"She's happy with God now. It's a blessing. God never gives us more than we can handle."

Instead, take your cues from the family and remember that their belief system might not be the same as yours.

Discounting Clichés

"I know just how you feel. Be glad you don't have problems like … At least you had 30 years together."

Instead, use phrases such as these: "*He sounds like he was a very special person.*" "*Let me sit with you for a while.*" "*Tell me how you are doing.*"

Children and Loss

Grieving family members may look to you for guidance regarding children. Children have three main questions when it comes to a death (Worden, 2001)—Did I cause the death? Is it going to happen to me? Who is going to take care of me?

Children should have the death explained in a straightforward manner. Avoid using euphemisms such as, "Grandpa has gone to sleep," or "We lost Uncle Bill today." Younger children especially are going to wonder why no one is trying to wake up Grandpa or find Uncle Bill. Encourage families to use simple explanations such as, "Grandpa died because he was very sick and his heart stopped beating." Keep in mind that expression of grief varies with a child's developmental stage (Worden, 2001).

In this time of great stress, children especially need to feel safe and cared for. Observe how the family is responding to any children present. If you are sensing disorganization among the family, you might help direct them by suggesting that one family member be designated to watch over the children.

Reassure families that children should be included in the grieving process as much as the child wants. Children and teens benefit from death rituals and traditions in the same way adults do (Myers, Norlander, & Young, 1999). Seeing the body can reinforce the reality of the death, and participating in rituals can provide personal meaning. However, take your clues from the family.

Self Care

Remember that nurses grieve too when patients die. Allow yourself time to honor the patient who has died and the work you did to care for that patient. A hospice nurse said of her own grief, "I cry with the family. I also try to take some quiet time—sometimes it's a short walk, sometimes I just sit in my car. But I need the time to remember that patient."

Just as families need to share the stories of their loved one, you might need to share stories with other staff. If you work in an institution or agency where you experience a lot of death, consider organizing a periodic memorial service to remember those you have cared for.

Summary

A guiding principle of nursing care at the end of life is the acknowledgement of grief. As a skilled clinician, you need to assess and intervene in family grieving. Provide a safe and comfortable place for the family to hear the news of the loss. Allow the family to be with the deceased. Acknowledge the death and recognize that grief is an ongoing process. As an advocate, make sure your institution has procedures in place to acknowledge the death in a caring and compassionate manner. As a guide, be *present* for the family. Listen to their stories and their concerns. Be aware of the special needs of grieving children. Last, but not least, acknowledge your own grief at the loss of a patient.

References

Emanuel L.L., von Gunten, C.F., & Ferris, F.D., eds. (1999). The education in palliative and end-of-life care (EPEC) curriculum, module 2: The EPEC project. The Robert Wood Johnson Foundation. Retrieved 3 November 2008 from http://www.epec.net/EPEC/Webpages/ph.cfm.

Meyer, C. (2000). In *On our own terms: Moyers on dying*. New York: Thirteen/WNET, p. 6.

Myers, R.N., Norlander, L., & Young, J. (1999). *Some things you may need to know when a loved one dies.* Minneapolis, MN: Allina Health System.

Worden, J.W. (2001). *Children and grief: when a parent dies.* New York: Guilford.

Worden, J.W. (1991). *Grief counseling and grief therapy: A handbook for the mental health practitioner*, second edition. New York: Springer.

Zerwekh, J.V. (2006). *Nursing care at the end of life: Palliative care for patients and families.* Philadelphia: F.A. Davis.

Other Resources

Books

Corr, C.A., Nabe, C.M., & Corr, D.M. (2008). *Death and dying, life and living.* Belmont, CA: Wadsworth Publishing.

Doka, K.J. (ed.) (2007). *Living with Grief: Before and After Death.* Washington, DC: Hospice Foundation of America.

Redfern, S. (2008). *The Grieving Garden: Living with the Death of a Child.* Charlottesville, VA: Hampton Roads Publishing.

Web Resources

Growth House. www.growthhouse.org. Provides a listing of books on bereavement and links to other information.

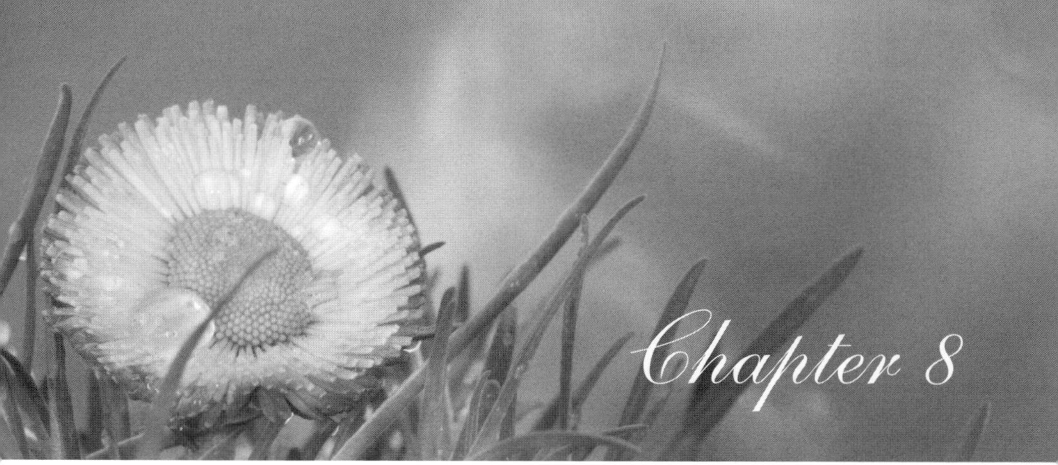

When a Child Is Dying

Pediatric End of Life

A circle no matter how small is still complete.

—Inscription on tombstone for Megan Zaihida Williams,
26 August 1991-13 December 1991

Children Die, Too

Mark is a 14-year-old with cystic fibrosis. He is currently hospitalized with a lung infection that is not responding to antibiotics. He has experienced a significant decline in the past 6 months with increased shortness of breath, fatigue, and weight loss. His mother has asked that no one talk with him about dying. One morning he asks his nurse, "Why won't anyone talk about how I want the rest of my life to go? I know I don't have much time left."

The nurse stops what she is doing and sits down at the bedside. She asks, "What would you like to have happen?"

Children are our symbol of life and hope. For children like Mark, dying is complicated by the fact that we believe in a certain order—children should grow up to have families, prosper, and live to be old. Medically, we treat children very aggressively to extend life. However, on a personal and familial level, we are often not honest with children. Caring for children like Mark is one of the biggest challenges you as a nurse can face. (See the sidebar "Differences Between Adult Care and Care of Dying Children.")

Differences between Adult Care and Care of Dying Children

- The developmental age of the child affects the understanding of treatments, the disease process, and death.
- Verbal skills might be limited, making pain and symptom assessment and management difficult.
- Many children receive very aggressive technological interventions in hopes of prolonging life and finding a cure.
- Often siblings are involved, and their care adds burden to stressed parents and family.
- Parents must make the ultimate decisions on treatment, which can be problematic if the child does not agree with the parent.

Nursing competence in caring for children begins with the understanding that, first and foremost, your patient is a child. Second, you are caring for a child who is dying. Caring for a child means understanding needs at different stages of development (Goldstein, Byrnes-Casey & Collins, 2005; Faulkner, 2008; Gibbons, 1993).

Infants and Toddlers

Children in this age category are learning to be separate from their primary caregivers. They particularly fear abandonment and separation. You need to provide close and physical contact and minimize separation from parents or primary caregivers. At this age, the concept of death is similar to that of temporary abandonment: "If I die, I'll come back tomorrow."

Preschoolers

At this stage, children are developing a sense of initiative. They fear loss of control, bodily injury, and being left alone. Concerning the concept of death, they have fantasy reasoning and magical thinking. Children in this age category often feel a great deal of guilt and responsibility for things they cannot explain. "If I had washed my hands like Mom said, I wouldn't be dying." Your use of simple concrete explanations is important.

School Age

At this stage, children begin developing logical thought and problem-solving ability. School-age children fear loss of control, the failure to live up to expectations of others, and death. They need to have their bodies treated with respect, to be offered specific factual information, and to have as much control over a situation as possible.

Adolescents

Children at this age are striving for their own sense of identity. They fear loss of control, altered body image, and separation from their peer group. They need honesty and the ability to make as many choices as possible.

With all children, good nursing skills equate to good communication skills. You need to ask three questions (Doka, 1996): What does the child need to know? What does the child want to know? What does the child understand?

Skilled Clinician: Assessing and Intervening in the Care of Children

Your assessment of pain and symptoms in children is often complicated by communication difficulties and a child's willingness to participate. Take into account the child's age and developmental stage. For example, most children over the age of 4 are capable of self-reporting pain (Goldstein, Byrnes-Casey & Collins, 2005; McGrath, 1990). However, you must tailor your language to the child's own vocabulary. For the child, pain might be called an "owie" or a "hurt."

You might find a dual assessment, one person asking the child and one asking the parents, to be helpful. For example, ask the child, "Do you tell others when you hurt?" At the same time, ask the parents, "Does your child tell others when he or she is hurting?"

When you are doing an assessment, keep in mind that children are easily distracted and often do not appear to be in distress. In one case, the parents reported that their child was not in pain because "he's sitting so quietly watching television." When the nurse explored this further, she discovered that he sat quietly because it hurt so much to move (Hilden, Watterson & Chrastek, 2000).

Sometimes children underreport a symptom because they are afraid of the treatment. For example, a 5-year-old refused to take his morphine tablets. The doctor used the child's favorite teddy bear to talk with the child. She discovered that the child refused the morphine because the tablets were too hard to swallow. She convinced the child to try liquid morphine because it might make his teddy bear feel better (Faulkner, 1997).

Children are more likely to talk about what is hurting or bothering them if they feel comfortable with the person who is talking to them. (See the sidebar "Tips for Talking with Children about Symptoms.")

Tips for Talking with Children about Symptoms

- Use language the child understands.
- Use play techniques such as puppets or art.
- Listen carefully to the child.
- Take your time with the child.

Pain

Treating pain in children is similar to treating pain in adults. You should use the analgesic pain ladder discussed in Chapter 3, beginning with mild analgesics such as acetaminophen and progressing to opioids. The preferred route of administration is oral. Often children have a permanent IV access, and parents are comfortable with giving meds through an IV. In these cases this route might be the best for both ease and pain relief. Most children do not like the rectal route. (Goldstein, Byrnes-Casey & Collins, 2005.)

Other Common Symptoms

Dying children experience the same array of distressing symptoms as adults: constipation, nausea and vomiting, anxiety, and sleep disturbances.

Anxiety is common in dying children. Your first step in approaching this symptom is to make sure that the anxiety is not caused by untreated pain. Providing reassurance and emotional support to both the child and the parents is often the most effective therapeutic approach (Hellsten & Kane, 2005; Miser & Miser, 1993).

Sleep disturbance can be particularly problematic because it is distressing for the child and exhausting for the parent. Medications can help, along with an exploration with the child of fears and anxiety that interfere with sleep (Hellsten & Kone 2005).

Active Dying

When death is near, your care involves preparing the family for what to expect. The dying process of a child is similar to that of an adult. Common signs to look for include the following:

- **Alertness and sleep changes:** You might see confusion, restlessness, and a decreased level of consciousness. Encourage the family to maintain gentle physical contact.
- **Breathing changes:** As with adults, a child's breathing might become very rapid, very shallow, and might include 10–30-second periods of no breathing. Sometimes oxygen can be comforting. Also, encourage the family to elevate the head of the bed. Assure the family that any gurgling sounds because of secretions are not causing the child discomfort.
- **Temperature changes:** As the child's heat-regulating system fails, his or her hands and feet can become cool. As in an adult, the child does not usually feel cold with this. You might also see an elevated temperature. Treat with cool washcloths.

Advocating for Children: Meeting the Needs of Both the Patient and the Family

Because the issues in caring for dying children are so multidimensional and complex, your nursing role as an advocate is critical in making sure that the needs of both the child and the family are met.

Communication Between Child and Family

One of your most difficult areas to address is communication between the child and the family. As mentioned earlier in the chapter, a dying child and his or her parents might not be in agreement with the course of care or treatment. Parents are often very protective and reluctant to talk openly with their child about the prognosis. Research has indicated, however, that children are very aware of their prognosis and want to be involved in the decision making. Much of the research done on communication with the dying child shows that families rarely regret sharing too much information but do regret sharing too little (Faulkner, 1993).

In advocating for clear communication between parent and child, use the resources of the health care team. If you assess the need, engage the physician, social worker, or chaplain. Many children's programs employ child life staff members who are trained to address the psychosocial needs of children at different developmental stages. They can also be a helpful resource.

In advocating for communication between the child and the family, also remember that the family includes siblings. Brothers and sisters can often feel left out during the strain and anxiety of a life-threatening illness. They should be included in family conferences and communications as much as possible. Again, you can find child life specialists to be of particular help in dealing with sibling issues.

Communications with the Parents

The serious illness of a child places enormous stress on parents. Studies indicate that the better informed parents are about their child's condition, the better they are able to participate meaningfully in care decisions (Hinds, Oakes, & Furman 2005). Your nursing advocacy includes understanding the needs of the parents and keeping parents well informed. Parents' priorities include honest and complete information, ready access to staff, communication and care coordination, emotional expression and support by staff, preservation of the parent-child relationship, and recognition of faith as an important support (Meyer, Ritholz, Burns & Truog, 2006).

Part of communication with parents is an ongoing assessment of their ability to understand and comprehend what is happening to their child. For example, the mother of a child with a brain tumor said, "Our nurse was incredibly helpful. She gave us information in terms we could understand. Sometimes, when we were overwhelmed, she'd say, 'I'm going to give you some time to absorb all this; then I'm coming back so we can talk again.'"

Effective communication with parents also means taking into account parents in nontraditional families. If the mother and father are divorced, for example, make sure everyone is informed. Use the skills of other team members such as social workers or chaplains to help facilitate communication in difficult family situations.

Communication with the Doctor

Communication with the doctor is crucial for the patient, family, and the rest of the health care team in dealing with a dying child. Researchers have found this to be a problem area. Parents who have lost a child often report that physician communication was vague and confusing. In addition, a survey of pediatric oncologists indicated that 47 percent do not initiate conversations about advance care planning, but instead wait for families to bring up the topic (Hilden et al., 2001).

Ways that you can advocate for clearer communications include the following:

- **Setting up family conferences that include the physician and other team members.**
- **Advocating for communication between physician specialists.** In one example, the nurse set up a telephone conference call for the family pediatrician, the pediatric oncologist, and the pediatric cardiologist to make sure the family was receiving a consistent message.
- **Clarifying in simple terminology the level of understanding the patient and family have during a conference with the physician.** Ask the question, "Can you tell me in your own words what Dr. X is saying about the chemotherapy?"

Sometimes families don't know what information to ask for. Advocating can also mean helping the family frame the questions for the physician. (See the sidebar "What Questions to Ask.")

What Questions to Ask

- How will the treatment help my child?
- What harm might we expect?
- What can you do with the information if we put our child through another test?
- Will the test change the course of treatment?

Care at Home

Studies have shown that most terminally ill children and their families do better when the child is cared for at home (Lauer, Mulhern, Schell & Camitta, 1989). As an advocate, especially for a hospitalized child, you need to ask the question not only of the physician, but also of the patient and family: "Can my patient go home?" If the answer is "yes," then you need to follow up with the health care team to make this possible. Make sure you know the community resources for home care and hospice for children.

Guiding Children and Families: Understanding the Needs of the Child

As a guide for your patient and for the family, model the behavior that s hows an understanding of the needs of the child. According to the National Hospice and Palliative Care Organization (2000) dying children need the following:

- **Love, security, and reassurance:** You can provide this through touch, play, and above all a willingness to listen to what the child says.
- **Honesty and information:** Communicate in terms of the child's world of understanding.
- **Control:** Even small choices such as what to eat or which color of medicine to take first can be important.
- **Privacy:** Children need time to be alone.

❖ **Acknowledgement of purpose in life:** Like adults, children want to leave a legacy. This might come in the form of artwork, audio or video, or written work.

In your role as guide, you need to stay with the family even if they make choices or take treatment paths with which you do not personally agree. Parents have to make the ultimate difficult decisions about their children. They are the ones who have to live on with those choices. You need to support them in doing what they feel is right.

Summary

Caring for a dying child is one of the most challenging roles a nurse can play. It requires an understanding of the developmental stage of the patient, the unique physiological needs of a growing child, and the complex needs of the family. Advocating for children involves promoting communication among the patient, family, and health care system. Finally, guiding in this context means knowing the needs of the patient and being present and supportive for the family.

References

Doka, K.J. (1996). The cruel paradox: Children who are living with life-threatening illnesses. In Corr, C.A., & Corr, D.M., (Eds.). *Handbook of Childhood Death and Bereavement.* New York: Springer, pp. 89–105.

Faulkner, K.W. (2008). Children's understanding of death. In Armstrong-Daily, A., and Zarbock, S., (Eds.). *Hospice Care for Children.* New York: Oxford University Press, pp. 9–23.

Faulkner, K.W. (1997). Talking about death with a dying child. *American Journal of Nursing.* 97(6): 64,66,68-69.

Gibbons, M.B. (1993). Psychosocial aspects of serious illness. In Armstrong-Dailey, A., and Zarbock, S., (Eds.). *Hospice Care for Children.* New York: Oxford University Press, pp. 60–74.

Goldstein, M.L., Byrnes-Casey, M., & Collins, J.J. (2005). Pediatric pain: Knowing the child before you. In: Ferrell, B.R., & Coyle, N. (Eds.). *Textbook of Palliative Nursing.* New York: Oxford University Press. Pp.991-1007.

Hellsten, M.B., & Kane, J. (2005). Symptom management in pediatric palliative care. In: Ferrell, B.R., & Coyle, N. (eds.) *Textbook of Palliative Nursing*. New York: Oxford University Press. pp. 895-908.

Hilden, J. et al. (2001). Attitudes and practices among pediatric oncologists regarding end of life care: Results of the 1998 American society of clinical oncology survey. *Journal of Clinical Oncology* 19(1): 205–212.

Hilden, J.M., Watterson, J., & Chrastek, J. (2000). Tell the children. *Journal of Clinical Oncology* 18(17): 3193–3195.

Hinds, P.S., Oakes, L., & Furman, W. (2005). End of life decision making in pediatric oncology. In Ferrell, B.R., & Coyle, N., eds. *Textbook of Palliative Nursing*. New York: Oxford University Press.

Lauer, M.E., Mulhern, R.K., Schell, M.J., & Camitta, B.M. (1989). Long term follow up of parental adjustment following a child's death at home or hospital. *Cancer* 63: 988–994.

McGrath, P.A., (Ed.). (1990). *Pain in children: Nature, assessment, and treatment.* New York: The Guilford Press.

Meyer, E.C., Ritholz, M.D., Burns, J.P., & Truog, R.D. (2006). Improving the quality of end-of-life care in pediatric intensive care unit: Parents' priorities and recommendations. *Pediatrics.* 117(3): pp. 649–657.

Miser, J.S., & Miser, A. W. (1993). Pain and symptom control in hospice care for children. In Armstrong-Daily, A., & Zarbock, S., eds. *Hospice Care for Children*. New York: Oxford University Press, pp. 22–59.

National Hospice and Palliative Care Organization (NHPCO). (2000). *Compendium of pediatric palliative care.* Alexandria, VA: NHPCO.

Other Resources

American Academy of Pediatrics (AAP). Statement on palliative care for children. http://aappolicy.aappublications.org/policy-statement/index.dtl

Children's Hospice International (CHI). www.chionline.org

Redfern, S., & Gilbert, S.K. (2008). *The grieving garden: Living with the death of a child*. Charlottesville, VA. Hampton Roads Publishing Company.

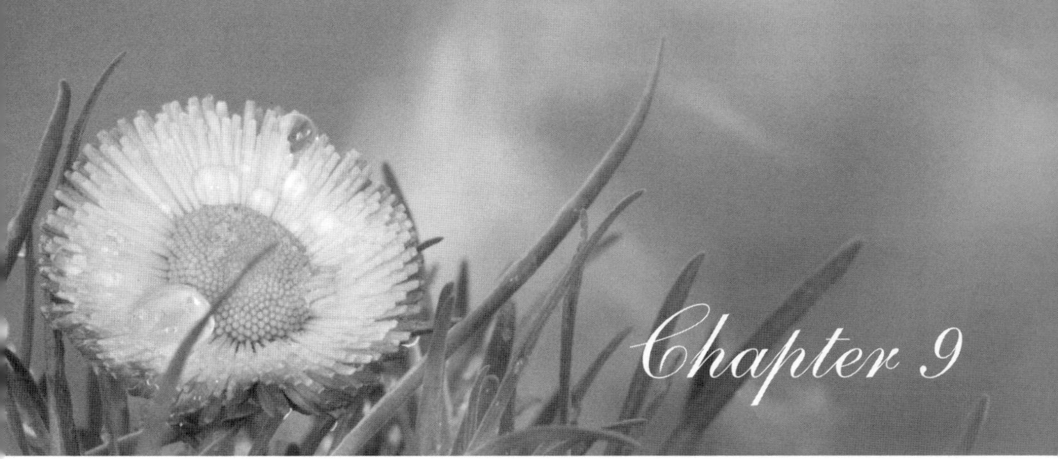

Cultural Sensitivity

Looking through Different Eyes

I may be forced to adopt a new way of life,
but my heart and spirit spring from the red earth.

—Painted Wolf (Doka and Davidson, 1998)

Making Room for Cultural Diversity

Mrs. Vang, a middle-aged Cambodian immigrant with advanced pancreatic cancer, is admitted to an oncology unit in extreme pain. Her family has not yet arrived at the hospital. When she is more comfortable, the doctor tries to talk with her about a "Do Not Resuscitate/Do Not Intubate" (DNR/DNI) status, but Mrs. Vang shakes her head. The oncology nurse sits down with her and says, "Please forgive me if I say anything that might be offensive to you. I'm trying to understand your needs so we can give you the best care possible."

Mrs. Vang nods and says, "I need my family first. Then we can make decisions."

In America, we live in a kaleidoscope of cultural, social, ethnic, and religious beliefs that influence how each person looks at dying. As nurses caring for dying patients, we need to acknowledge that our view of death and dying might be very different from that of our patients and their families.

For example, American medical practices place a high value on the concept of individual patient autonomy and the patient's right to know about his or her diagnosis. We stress the importance of communicating directly with patients and of telling them the diagnosis. In other countries that might not be the case (Koenig & Gates-Williams, 1995).

With our emphasis on the importance of individual rights, we expect patients to make their own decisions on treatment options. Yet, in many cultural groups, decision making is a group or family process (Sherman, 2005). Consider the mounting frustration of a hospice nurse caring for an immigrant patient from Southeast Asia. The patient was in extreme pain. In a discussion with her supervisor about the patient's uncontrolled pain, the nurse said, "I keep telling the wife to give him morphine on a regular basis. I don't know why she won't listen to me." With further exploration, the nurse discovered that the wife was not the primary decision maker in this situation. The elders of the family directed the patient's care. After the nurse spoke with the elders about the patient's pain and they agreed with her suggestions, the wife was able to start giving the morphine on a regular basis.

Our health care system is based on a scientific biomedical model of disease. Many other cultures have a more spiritual or nature-based view. For example, some Native Americans see illness as an imbalance between the heart, mind, body, and soul. Rather than looking for pharmaceutical or surgical remedies, they might look instead to a spiritual healer (Showalter, 1998).

Others might view our system with mistrust because of past or current experience. For example, the United States health care system has historically provided less access to health care for African-American communities in comparison to the White population. African-Americans are more likely to regard the withholding of aggressive treatment and advance directive planning with suspicion. (Hallenbeck, 2001).

Many of the culturally diverse patients and families we care for at the end of life have the added stressors of limited financial resources and health coverage. Culturally sensitive care includes taking these issues into consideration.

Understand Your Own Beliefs

In the previous situation with the nurse who encountered difficulties relieving her patient's pain, the nurse also discovered that she carried her own values and beliefs into the home. As she later told her supervisor, "It made me angry that the wife couldn't make decisions for herself." When you are looking at culturally sensitive care for dying patients, look at your own attitudes, beliefs, and practices. A number of cultural self-assessment tools exist that can help you better understand your own beliefs. (See the sidebar "Questions To Ask Yourself about Your Own Attitudes and Beliefs" and Web References at the end of this chapter for more self-assessment resources.)

Questions To Ask Yourself about Your Own Attitudes and Beliefs

- ❖ How was death talked about in your family?
- ❖ What kind of death would you prefer?
- ❖ What do you believe causes most deaths?
- ❖ If you were diagnosed with a terminal disease, would you want to be told?
- ❖ What efforts should be made to keep a seriously ill person alive?
- ❖ What do you consider a "good death"?

(DeSpelder, 1998)

The ability to know yourself can give you insight on how you might respond to someone whose answers are different from your own. For example, if you feel strongly about the importance of disclosure in the case of a terminal illness, you know you need to step back and listen carefully to the family that requests that a patient not be told of the diagnosis.

As another example, you might believe that a "good death" means dying peacefully at home surrounded by family. However, this is not a universal concept. Some Chinese immigrants choose to avoid death at home because they believe that the ghost of the person who died will inhabit the home (Koenig & Gates-Williams, 1995). Also, some African-Americans prefer end of life care in an intensive care unit, hospice residence, or long-term care facility so they will not be a burden to their families. (Duffy, Jackson, Schim, Ronis & Fowler, 2006a, 2006b).

Listen to the Patients

With the variety and complexity of cultural differences within our society, you can't *know* everything about each patient's beliefs and needs. The best approach you can take is one of honesty and active listening. It is okay to say, "I do not know much about your culture and beliefs, but I want to learn from you so I can give you the best care possible."

Several approaches can help you to be an effective listener:

- **Ask open-ended questions rather than questions that can be answered "yes" or "no."** This allows for discussion. For example, ask, "Tell me how you slept last night" instead of asking, "Did you sleep well last night?"
- **Be patient**. Sometimes a seemingly roundabout response to a question can yield valuable information.
- **Acknowledge the patient's perception of the illness**. If a patient says, "I believe a bad spirit has gotten into my stomach," try, "Tell me more about it," instead of saying, "No, it's a bacterial infection."

Listening to patients also means paying close attention to nonverbal communication. This includes facial expressions, eye contact, and touch. Evidence exists that facial expressions of emotions are universal (Andrews & Boyle, 2007). If a patient appears to be in distress, take that as a cue that he or she *is* in distress. You can validate your observation by simply saying, "You look sad or uncomfortable or in pain."

Eye contact can be a misinterpreted nonverbal signal. In European-American society, it is the accepted practice to make direct eye contact when you look at people. However, in some Asian and Native American cultures, it is considered disrespectful to look directly at a person you consider a superior. This could easily be misinterpreted in our culture as someone who is either not listening or not interested. If you are talking with a patient or family and they are not looking directly at you, clarify by asking "Do you understand what I am saying?"

Because touch has a wide variety of meanings, it is always reasonable to ask, for example, "Is it all right if I hold your hand, or hug you, or stroke your forehead?" Not all people welcome human touch. For example, some Asian cultures believe that strength resides in a person's head; to touch the head is a sign of great disrespect (Andrews & Boyle, 2007).

Avoid Stereotyping and Making Assumptions

No magical formula exists for understanding various cultures. Culture is not homogenous, and you can find a great deal of diversity among individuals even in the smallest cultural group. Beware of stereotyping or making assumptions based on general knowledge of a patient's culture rather than on a specific knowledge of the patient. For example, because you know that certain Asian cultures believe that patients should not be told of a terminal diagnosis, this does not mean you should assume that all Asian patients feel this way. You need to ask. "How much would you like to know about your illness?" (See the sidebar "Ways to Avoid Cultural Stereotyping.")

Ways To Avoid Cultural Stereotyping

- Prepare the patient for your questions by saying, "I am not very familiar with your customs. Please tell me if I ask questions that are offensive to you."
- Ask open-ended questions. Ask, "Who else would you like to have here while I talk with you?" instead of "Do you want your family here while I talk with you?" is a good question.
- Ask patients and families to help you identify resources that can enhance your understanding of their care needs: "Who in your community could help me better understand how to best care for you?" is a good question.

Use Trained Medical Interpreters

Caring for patients when you encounter a language barrier is one of the most challenging aspects of working with a culturally diverse population. You should engage trained medical interpreters whenever possible. Do not use family members or people who are not trained in medical interpretation unless it is absolutely necessary. Children in immigrant families often learn English before parents or grandparents and are asked to interpret. Not only are they not trained in medical language, but asking them to interpret places a heavy and sometimes embarrassing burden of responsibility on them. As one teenage boy said, "How could I ask my grandmother about the private parts of her body?"

When using trained interpreters, consider the following suggestions (Howard, 2008):

- Prepare the interpreter ahead of time that you will be discussing end of life issues or using the word "dying."
- Position yourself at eye-level with the patient and speak to the patient, not the interpreter.
- Keep sentences and questions concise.
- Following the interview, give the interpreter a chance to process the interview and ask you questions.

In reality, you will not always find it possible to use a trained medical interpreter. If you must communicate with a patient or family without the aid of an interpreter, do not raise your voice. Speak in a low, moderate voice using a polite and formal tone. You can also try the following:

- **Use simple words:** Instead of discomfort, use *pain.*
- **Ask direct questions:** Ask questions such as "*Are you in pain?*"
- **Give instructions in simple language and demonstrate them:** "Put the medicine into the dropper like this. Then place it in his cheek like this."
- **Discuss one topic at a time:** For example, do not ask, "Are you having trouble breathing or sleeping at night?"

Whenever possible, identify resources to help you with the language barrier. Look for materials written in the patient's language. Find someone in the community who can help you with simple phrases.

Use Community Resources

Many communities of diversity have their own "cultural informants." These are people from within the community who interact with the larger American society. Cultural informants can be invaluable both to help you better understand the needs of your patient and to help you link the patient with community programs.

Advocating for Patients and Families

If you work in a health care institution, look at the policies of your workplace regarding cultural sensitivity. Do you have trained interpreters available? Do you have written resources for your patients in their own language? Are your policies flexible enough to accommodate patients and families of diverse backgrounds?

To work toward a culturally supportive place for patients and families to be at the end of life consider the following:

- **Create space to accommodate extended families.**
- **Institute nonrestrictive visiting hours.** An Asian-American daughter said of her mother's death, "In my family, we do not believe people should die alone. When my mother was in the hospital, they made us go home for the night. She died alone. They said that when they found her, she had tears in her eyes. I will live with that always."
- **Allow important rituals such as traditional healing ceremonies.**

At death, ask how the family prefers the body to be treated. Funeral rituals and rites vary with culture and religion. For example (Zerwekh, 2006; Ealing Council, 2004):

- In the Jewish tradition, burial should occur within 24 hours of the death. The body should not be left unattended.
- In the Muslim tradition, the burial should occur before noon on the day of the death. The body should be buried with the head towards Mecca.
- In the Buddhist tradition, the family stays with and prepares the body. Death is considered a prelude to existence in another state.
- In the Hindu tradition, cremation should occur within 24 hours.
- In Western Christian tradition, the funeral industry is relied upon to prepare the body and organize the rituals.

Summary

Working with patients and families of different cultural, ethnic, religious, and socio-economic backgrounds during the last steps of a journey in life is an art. It's the art of being aware of diverse needs, the art of listening, and the art of balancing your own culture and the culture of your institution with the culture of the patient and family.

References

Andrews, M.A., & Boyle, J.S. (2007). *Transcultural concepts of nursing care (5th ed.)*. Philadelphia, PA: Lippincott Williams and Wilkens.

DeSpelder, L.A. (1998). Developing cultural competency. In Doka, K.J., & Davidson, J.D. *Living with Grief.* Washington, DC: Hospice Foundation of America, pp. 97–106.

Doka, K.J., & Davidson, J.D. (1998). *Living with grief when illness is prolonged*. Washington, DC: Hospice Foundation of America,

Duffy, S., Jackson, F., Schim, S., Ronis, D., & Fowler, K. (2006a). Cultural concepts at the end of life. *Nursing Older People,* 18(8), 10-14.

Duffy, S., Jackson, F., Schim, S., Ronis, D., & Fowler, K.E. (2006b). *Journal of the American Geriatrics Society,* 54(1), 150-157.

Ealing Council (2004). *Funeral rites across different cultures.* Retrieved 16 October 2008 from http://www.egfl.org.uk/export/sites/egfl/categories/teaching/curriculum/subjects/re/_articles_docs/Furneral_Rites_website.doc

Hallenbeck, J.L. (2001). Intercultural differences and communication at the end of life. *Primary Care,* 28(2), 401-413.

Howard, S. (2008.) Fast fact and concept #154: Use of interpreters in palliative care. www.eperc.mcw.edu/fastFact/ff_154.htm. Accessed 10/11/2008.

Koenig, B., & Gates-Williams, J. (1995). Understanding cultural difference in caring for dying patients. *Western Journal of Medicine* 163(3): 244–248.

Sherman, D.W. (2005). Spiritually and culturally competent palliative care. In Matzo, M.L., and Sherman, D.W., (Eds.). *Palliative Care Nursing: Quality Care to the End of Life, 2nd edition*. New York: Springer.

Showalter, S.E. (1998). Looking through different eyes: Beyond cultural diversity. In Doka, K.J., and Davidson, J.D. *Living with Grief.* Washington, DC: Hospice Foundation of America, pp. 71–82.

Zerwekh, J.V. (2006). *Nursing care at the end of life: Palliative care for patients and families.* Philadelphia: F.A. Davis.

Other Resources

Books

Geissler, E.M. (2007). *Mosby's pocket guide to cultural assessment.* St. Louis, MO: Mosby.

Lipson, J.G., & Dibble, S.L., eds. (2005). *Culture and clinical care.* San Francisco: UCSF Nursing Press.

Web Sites

Office of Minority Health Resource Center. Washington, DC: Department of Health and Human Services. Includes National Standards on Culturally and Linguistically Appropriate Services. Retrieved 11 October 2008. www.omhrc.gov

Oncology Nursing Society Multicultural Toolkit. Learning kit for providing culturally competent care to patients. Retrieved 11 October 2008. http://www.ons.org/clinical/Special/toolkit.shtml

Self assessment, an essential aspect of culturally competent care. Self assessment tools for health care providers. Retrieved 11 October 2008. http://www11.georgetown.edu/research/gucchd/nccc/foundations/assessment.html

United States Department of Health and Human Services. Nursing modules for culturally competent care. Retrieved 11 October 2008. http://www.thinkculturalhealth.org

Chapter 10

Hospice

Hospice adds life to days when days can no longer be added to life.

—*The Family Handbook of Hospice Care*
(Fairview Health Services, 1999)

A Philosophy of Care

George is a 78-year-old man who lives in a senior citizens' high-rise with his 76-year-old wife. He suffered a severe stroke 5 days ago. He is currently hospitalized on a neurology floor and is minimally responsive. His wife and family have chosen not to pursue any further aggressive treatment for him, including the insertion of a feeding tube. The family asks the nurse, "What do we do now?"

She says, "What do you know about hospice care?"

The wife looks concerned and says, "But George didn't want to be put someplace. He always wanted to be at home." The nurse then explains that hospice can help the family take George home and care for him there. The nurse discusses the family preference to care for the patient at home with the physician and obtains an order for hospice care. The nurse then arranges a conference with the family, the social worker, and a hospice coordinator to discuss discharge plans.

To explain hospice to your patients and families, you need to understand the basic philosophy of hospice care. The focus of hospice is on ensuring that a patient's remaining days are comfortable. It is considered the gold standard of care for people at the end of life's journey. (See the sidebar "Hospice Care.")

Hospice Care

- Emphasizes living as fully as possible
- Provides relief from the physical, emotional, and spiritual distress that often accompany a life-limiting illness
- Provides support for the family while they are caring for their loved one
- Provides grief support for the family following the death

Most patients enrolled in hospice are able to spend their final days in the comfort of their own home. For those who cannot be at home, hospice care can be provided in a hospital, long-term care facility, or other type of residential setting.

The hospice philosophy of care embraces a holistic approach to the patient and family. The focus of care is on comfort and dignity for the patient and family during the last months, weeks, and days of the patient's life.

Who Qualifies for Hospice Care?

Hospice care is provided for patients who have a terminal diagnosis and are no longer pursuing active aggressive treatment to cure the disease. Most hospice programs use admission criteria established through the Hospice Medicare Benefit. To receive services patients need to have a diagnosis with a prognosis of 6 months or less as certified by a physician. This means that given the patient's disease and current status, the doctor expects that he or she is going to die within 6 months. Patients also need to sign a hospice consent form agreeing to accept care that focuses on comfort rather than on either cure or treatments to prolong life.

Referral to hospice does not require a physician's order. However, a physician must be involved after a plan of care for the patient has been established.

The 6-Month Prognosis

The 6-month prognosis can sometimes be a barrier for referral to hospice. Physicians can be reluctant to predict that a patient is going to die in this period of time. If you feel a patient could benefit from hospice care, and the physician is unsure of the prognosis, remember, this time frame is only an estimate. According to information released by the National Hospice and Palliative Care Organization (NHPCO) in 2007, whereas most patients enrolled in hospice live less than 2 months, some continue to receive services much longer than 6 months. The hospice program reevaluates the patient on a regular basis. Research has shown that physicians are more likely to overestimate a lifespan than underestimate it (Christakis & Lamont, 2000). Consider approaching a reluctant physician with these two questions: Would you be surprised if this patient was still alive in 6 months? Is this patient sick enough to die?

Hospice Philosophy of Care

The second criterion for hospice admission, the patient's agreeing to a hospice philosophy of care, can also be problematic. Hospices interpret the meaning of this differently. For example, some hospice programs do not admit patients who are receiving chemotherapy because they view this treatment as curative rather than palliative. If your patient is receiving specialized treatments, discuss these treatments with the hospice admissions coordinator. If one program does not accept a patient, try another.

How Do I Approach Patients and Families about Hospice Care?

Patients who accept hospice care have crossed a difficult bridge from looking to medical care for cure or for life extension to looking at life completion. Talking about hospice is not an easy conversation. The best approach is an honest one: "It looks like the course of your care is changing. I'd like to talk with you about hospice." Some patients and families are going to be willing and interested to learn more. Others need time. And still others do not want to consider hospice as an option. Listen carefully to questions the patients and families have and provide as much information as they want. You should also consider this a good time to engage other members of the team, including the physician, social worker, and chaplain.

You are going to find common concerns patients and their families have when talking about hospice, including the following:

- "Are you sure its time to talk about hospice? Can't we try some other treatments?" Review with the patient and family their understanding of the illness and the treatment options. Use simple and straightforward language to clarify their questions. Patients receiving hospice care still have many treatment options available to them.
- "If we talk about hospice, the patient might give up hope." Clarify what is meant by *hope*. For the seriously ill, hope can take on a dimension very different than one of cure. Hope to them might mean having the time to accomplish some goals such as saying good-bye or putting their affairs in order. For some, hope means being at home. For others, hope is defined by feeling comforted and cared for.
- "Does this mean the doctor is going to quit treating me?" Many patients feel they are going to be abandoned by their physicians if they agree to hospice care. Avoid saying, "We can do nothing more for you." Instead, reassure patients that their physician is going to continue to give direct care. Also assure them that many treatments still exist and are going to be used, but now the focus is going to be on comfort and palliation, not cure.

The Hospice Medicare Benefit

Hospice care is covered under a special Medicare benefit. It is also provided under Medicaid and private insurance companies. The Medicare Hospice Benefit currently covers the following:

- **Medical and symptom management focused on enhancing comfort:** Care is provided by a team of professionals including the patient's primary physician, nurses, and the hospice medical director.
- **Emotional and spiritual care:** Hospice care includes visits by social workers, chaplains, and volunteers.
- **Coverage for medications, supplies, and medical equipment related to the terminal diagnosis**
- **Assistance with bathing, personal care, and homemaking**
- **Volunteer services for respite, companionship, and errands**
- **Hospitalization for acute episodes and extended hours of care in the home for acute episodes**
- **Respite care for times when the family is exhausted or unable to provide care**
- **Grief support for the family**

In George's case, which was discussed at the beginning of the chapter, the hospice staff can help arrange for his discharge to home. This can include ordering a hospital bed and any other equipment the family might need to care for him in his apartment. He is going to receive regular visits from the hospice nurse to manage his physical care. A home health aide can help with George's bath and personal care. The hospice social worker can help his wife and family deal with some of the complexities of caring for a person at home. In addition, the hospice chaplain is available to discuss spiritual issues. Hospice volunteers are also available to provide companionship and respite care or to run errands.

Hospice provides the family with 24-hour call service. George is also eligible for extended hours of care during a medical crisis. The goal of his care is to provide the support George and his family need to keep him comfortable and in his apartment as long as possible. When George dies, the hospice program follows up with his family, providing support and counseling up to 13 months after the death.

While hospice care under the Hospice Medicare Benefit is a comprehensive benefit, it does have limitations. You need to be aware of those areas not covered under the benefit. (See the sidebar "Hospice Medicare Benefit Limitations.")

Hospice Medicare Benefit Limitations

- Does not provide 24-hour caregiving services.
- Provides extended hours of care (continuous care) only during a crisis. If a patient routinely needs 24-hour care that the family is unable to provide, the hospice social worker can assist the family in establishing services. These are generally private pay arrangements.
- Does not cover treatments and medications unrelated to the terminal illness. For example, if a patient is diabetic and insulin dependent, but the terminal diagnosis is lung cancer, hospice does not cover the cost of the insulin and related supplies.
- Does not cover curative or experimental treatments aimed at cure.

Advocating for Your Patients

When facing a life-limiting or terminal illness, most patients prefer to be cared for in their own home. As an advocate, ask the patient and family, "Where would you like to be?" Hospice is a comprehensive program covered by insurance and Medicare that strives to keep patients in their own home as long as possible. Make sure you are aware of the hospice programs in your area. Have brochures and information available to your patients and families. Offer hospice care as an option. One of the most common comments hospice administrators receive from family surveys is the wish that hospice had been offered sooner.

Summary

Hospice care is a philosophy of care that encompasses the complex physical, personal, familial, and spiritual needs of a dying person. Care is provided by a team of health professionals including the patient's primary physician, a hospice nurse, social worker, chaplain, home health aides, volunteers, and others as needed. Under the Hospice Medicare Benefit, patients qualify for hospice if they have a terminal illness with a prognosis of 6 months or less and if they choose a philosophy of care that emphasizes comfort over cure.

References

Christakis, N.A., & Lamont, E.B. (2000). Extent and determinants of error in doctors' prognosis in terminally ill patients: Prospective cohort study. *British Medical Journal* 320 (7233): 469–472.

Fairview Health Services. (1999). *The Family Handbook of Hospice Care.* Minneapolis, MN: Fairview Press.

National Hospice and Palliative Care Organization (NHPCO). (2007). NHPCO facts and figures: Hospice care in America. Retrieved 12 October 2008. http://www.nhpco.org/files/public/Statistics_Research/NHPCO_facts-and-figures_Nov2007.pdf

Other Resources

Lattanzi-Licht, M., Mahoney, J., & Miller, G. (1998). *The hospice choice: In pursuit of a peaceful death.* New York: Fireside Books.

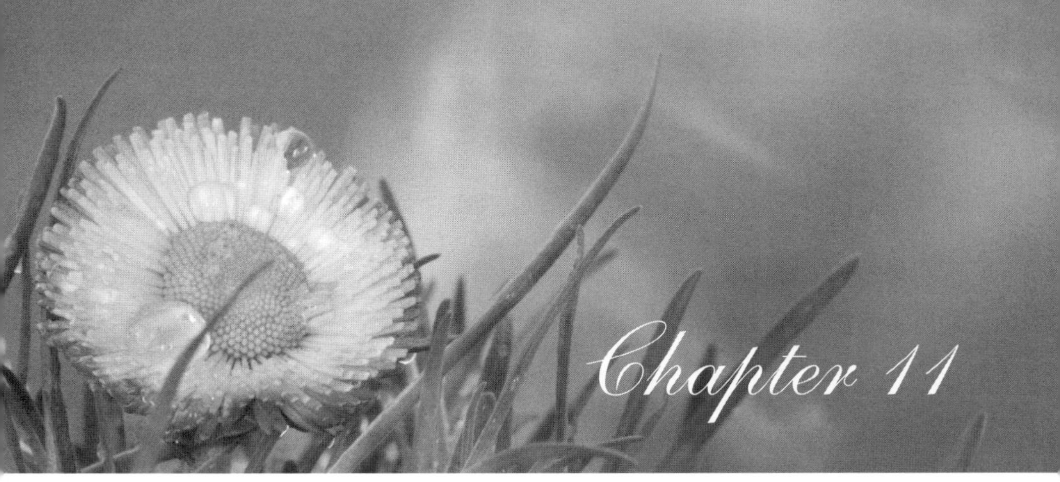

Ethical Issues in End-of-Life Care

It is often exquisitely difficult to determine what the right response is when a terminally ill and suffering patient pleads with you to help speed her dying.

—Judith Kennedy Schwarz (2005)

Stacy is a 47- year-old woman with advanced breast cancer and metastases to the lung and brain. She suffered a respiratory arrest during a surgical procedure 4 days ago. She was resuscitated and is currently in the intensive care unit on a ventilator, unable to speak for herself. Her husband, Tom, has talked with the nurse about wanting "everything done" for her. Her mother, Edith, has told the nurse in a separate conversation that she and Tom do not agree on Stacy's care and that she wants to stop aggressive treatment and take her daughter off all the "machines." To discuss the next steps in Stacy's care, the nurse calls a family conference that includes Tom, Edith, the hospital rounding physician who is managing the care, and the hospital chaplain.

The generations alive today are the first to live in an era of advanced medical technology like ventilators, cardiopulmonary resuscitation (CPR), and tube feedings that can prolong life and delay death (Dunn, 2002). Patients and families are faced with difficult choices, and nursing is often at the center of these difficult situations. Decisions become even more complex when the patients cannot speak for themselves and families are conflicted. A fast-paced medical system that often responds to an immediate crisis without having the time to take into consideration a patient's long-term needs or goals can add to this difficulty.

Stacy's family needs to explore a number of issues in determining her care. Does she have an advance directive that indicates her wishes in this situation? Did she ever discuss what she might want with her family? If not, then using an ethical framework can help the family in making difficult and often contentious decisions.

Health Care Ethics

Health care ethics (also called bioethics or medical ethics) is the "study of moral obligations of health care providers and society in preventing and treating disease and injury and in caring for people with illness and injury." (Berry, 2005, p.263).

The most common health care ethics framework is based on four principles (Butts & Rich, 2007).

- **Beneficence:** Beneficence is the obligation to act for another's benefit. In end-of-life care, this means looking at the benefits and burdens of a particular action or treatment. For example, is the treatment going to relieve pain and suffering but place a heavy burden on the family trying to care for the patient at home?
- **Nonmaleficence:** Nonmaleficence is the obligation to "do no harm." In end-of-life care, it involves looking at the harm a treatment or course of action might cause. Is the treatment going to prolong the patient's dying without increasing quality or comfort?
- **Autonomy:** Autonomy is based on a person's right to choose independently. In end-of-life care, the right to choose also means the right to refuse treatment.
- **Justice:** Justice encompasses fair and equitable treatment. It can also have a broader meaning in looking at the best use of limited resources.

Common Ethical Dilemmas and Conflicts

You face ethical dilemmas when you encounter conflict or when controversy exists over a treatment or course of action. Often you find these conflicts occurring when a patient lacks the capacity to make decisions for him- or herself, does not have an advance directive, or has not communicated his or her wishes to family members or care providers prior to losing capacity. Decision-making capacity refers to the ability of a patient to understand a proposed course of treatment including the benefits and burdens and to communicate treatment preferences or wishes to others (Schwarz, 2005). See the sidebar "Assessing Decision-Making Capacity."

Assessing Decision-Making Capacity

Questions you should ask the patient:

- Can you tell me why your doctor is recommending this treatment?
- Can you tell me what the recommended treatment is?
- Can you tell me about the benefits and risks of this treatment?

(Adapted from Schwarz, 2005)

Many of the common dilemmas in end-of-life care for patients and families involve either starting a treatment or discontinuing it.

- **Resuscitation:** Should CPR be attempted if a patient's heart stops or he or she stops breathing?
- **Artificial nutrition and hydration:** Should IV hydration or tube feedings be initiated, or if initiated, discontinued?
- **Ventilator support:** Should a patient be placed on a ventilator, or if the patient is already on one, should it be discontinued?
- **Initiation of treatment such as surgery or chemotherapy that might be considered futile or of no benefit to the patient**

Dilemmas also arise over use of medications such as opioids or sedatives to control pain and other symptoms. Of special concern here is the principle of *double effect*. Can the treatment, such as high doses of morphine, while relieving the pain, cause side effects such as respiratory depression that hasten death? If you use an ethical framework to address these issues, you need to meet several conditions (Zerwekh, 2006):

- The act must not be intrinsically wrong (that is, medications are not intentionally given in order to cause the death).
- The intention must be to do good (that is, to relieve the pain).
- The good effect must outweigh the bad effect (that is, relief of suffering versus a shortened life.)

One of the most controversial discussions in the past two decades centers on the provision of aid in dying by the medical profession. *Physician-assisted suicide* or *physician aid in dying* refers to the physician prescribing lethal dosages of medication that the patient can take. Physician aid in dying is legal in only one state, Oregon, and is available only to terminally ill patients who are considered competent to make this choice and have been evaluated for depression. (*See* http://www.oregon.gov/DHS/ph/pas for more information on the Death With Dignity Act.)

In contrast to physician-assisted suicide, where the patient takes his or her own life, *euthanasia* refers to the killing of a patient with "merciful intent." Euthanasia is not legal and is condemned by most ethicists (Zerwekh, 2006). The Hospice and Palliative Nurses Association's (HPNA) code of ethics states opposition to involvement in either physician-assisted suicide or active euthanasia (HPNA, 2005).

Role of the Skilled Clinician in Difficult Decisions

As a skilled clinician, you have several roles in caring for your patients and their families. The first is to have a thorough understanding of the patient's illness, including the treatment options, implications of treatment, and usual progression of the course of the illness. For example, John is a 56-year-old man diagnosed with amyotrophic lateral sclerosis (ALS) three years ago. Since that time, he has lost his ability to walk and has recently experienced more difficulty breathing and managing his secretions. He is nearing the point in his illness where he has to choose whether or not to go on a ventilator.

You can help John and his family with this decision by providing honest and factual information about the expected course of ALS. You can also help John and his family identify the possible treatment options and the implications of those options. Do they understand the care needs involved with a ventilator-dependent patient, very likely with a tracheostomy? Do they understand the possible harm or discomfort a ventilator could cause and the future decisions regarding stopping the ventilator? Do they understand their resources if they make this choice? Do they understand the implications if they choose not to have the ventilator? (See the sidebar "Gathering Relevant Information.")

Gathering Relevant Information

Questions you should ask:

- Does this patient have decision-making capacity? If not, who is the surrogate decision-maker?
- Has the patient expressed his or her wishes before losing capacity, either verbally or in a written advance directive?
- What are the choices that need to be addressed?
- Who are the relevant family members or stakeholders in this decision?

Your use of the interdisciplinary team is a key component in helping patients and families sort through difficult decisions. Most decisions are neither simple nor black and white, and you must take into consideration not only the physical implications but also a lifetime of values and beliefs of both the patient and the family.

Advocate: Making Sure Wishes Are Honored

In times of difficult decisions, patients, families, and health care providers are not always united. You can play a vital role in advocating for the wishes of the patient.

Kristin, a palliative care nurse in a hospital, related the time she sat with a family to talk about their elderly mother who was unresponsive following a stroke. Of the three daughters, two wanted comfort care for their mother, and the third insisted that a feeding tube be placed: "If we don't, I feel like we're killing Mom."

The patient had a written advance directive that clearly stated that she did not want a feeding tube. Kristin was able to convey this to the daughter in a gentle but firm manner, "You are fortunate that you don't have to make this decision because your mother already has."

As a nurse you might find yourself in a situation where advocating for the patient conflicts with the advice of another health care professional. For example, Margaret, a hospice nurse, was caring for a patient in his late 60s with severe diabetes and heart failure. The patient developed gangrene in his toes and was too ill to participate in decision-making. His physician recommended an amputation, but Margaret knew the patient had specifically stated he wanted to die with his body intact. Unfortunately, the patient did not have a written advance directive, and the patient's wife was too upset to disagree with the doctor who told her he would die without the amputation.

In this case, Margaret, as the advocate, had to take a risk in contradicting the physician's recommendations. With the help of the social worker, she brought the family, including the wife and the children, in to talk about what everyone thought the patient would want. They were able to decide on comfort measures rather than the amputation. The patient was discharged to a comfort care unit and died peacefully.

Guide

Often the most important role you can play involves guiding patients and families to make decisions that are consistent with their values and beliefs. By reframing the discussion and questions back to the concepts of benefit versus burden, harm versus good, respect for autonomy and consideration of justice, you can provide the guidance they might need.

For example, in the case of the patient who faced amputation, you might ask the following questions:

- What is the amputation going to do for the quality of the patient's life? Is it going to extend life or relieve painful symptoms? Allow time for the family to accept the terminal status.

- ❖ What harm might the amputation do: loss of body image? painful surgery with poor recovery?
- ❖ Does this surgery conflict with the patient's values or wishes?

What about a Nurse's Personal Ethics, Beliefs, and Values?

Because decisions at the end of life entail moral, ethical, and even spiritual values, you might find your own values in conflict with the wishes of the patient, the family, or the other health care providers. You can be in the position of discontinuing treatments, administering medications, or initiating treatments you believe are wrong or harmful. Under these circumstances you need to step back and separate your own personal values from the situation. Try to understand the meaning of the illness to the patient and family. You can enlist the help of the interdisciplinary team available to you. Perhaps the physician, chaplain, social worker, or other team members can help you work through the issues.

Most hospitals and institutions have ethics committees. These committees are usually interdisciplinary and use an ethical framework to discuss and analyze the dilemma. Ethics committees can often provide recommendations and guidance, and you should view them as another good resource for you.

Ethics and Culture

The bioethic framework discussed in this chapter generally reflects European-American values. Other cultures have different perspectives, and these must be taken into consideration in issues of end-of-life decision making. For example, as Sherman (2005) notes, within many non-European-American cultures, the community and family members make decisions rather than the individuals. They find the concept of autonomy foreign and confusing. In other cultures, full disclosure to the patient is considered disrespectful.

Summary

Ethics in end-of life-care encompasses the moral obligation to care for a patient in a way that prevents harm and benefits the patient. As a patient nears the end of life, he or she and his or her family face many difficult decisions regarding starting and discontinuing treatments. As a skilled clinician, you should have a good understanding of the illness and be able to communicate this knowledge artfully and truthfully to the patient and family. As an advocate, you need to ensure that the patient's wishes are heard, understood, and honored. As a guide, your communication skills are essential in walking patients and families through these difficult decisions.

References

Berry, P. (ed.) (2005). *Core curriculum for the generalist hospice and palliative nurse, Second edition.* Dubuque, Iowa: Kendell/Hunt.

Butts, J.B. & Rich, K.L. (2007), *Nursing ethics: Across the curriculum and into practice, Second revised edition.* Boston: Jones and Bartlett.

Dunn, H. (2002). *Hard choices for loving people: CPR, artificial feeding, comfort care and the patient with a life-threatening illness, Fourth edition.* Herdon, VA: A & A Publishers. www.hardchoices.com

Hospice and Palliative Nurses Association. (2005). Guiding Principles. Retrieved 14 October 2008 from http://www.hpna.org/DisplayPage.aspx?Title=Guiding%20Principles

Schwarz, J. (2005). Ethical aspects of palliative care. In Matzo, M. L., and Sherman, D.W., eds. *Palliative Care Nursing: Quality Care to the End of Life 2nd Edition.* New York: Springer, pp. 151–183.

Sherman, D.W. (2005). Spirituality and culture as domains of quality palliative care. In Matzo, M.L., & Sherman, D.W., eds. *Palliative care nursing: Quality care to the end of life Second Edition.* New York, Springer: pp. 3–45.

Zerwekh, J.V. (2006). *Nursing care at the end of life: Palliative care for patients and families.* Philadelphia: F. A. Davis, pp. 179–211.

Other Resources

American Medical Association's Statement on End-of-Life Care.
http://www.ama-assn.org/ama/pub/category/7567.html

American Nurses Association Code of Ethics.
http://nursingworld.org/ethics/code/protected_nwcoe813.htm

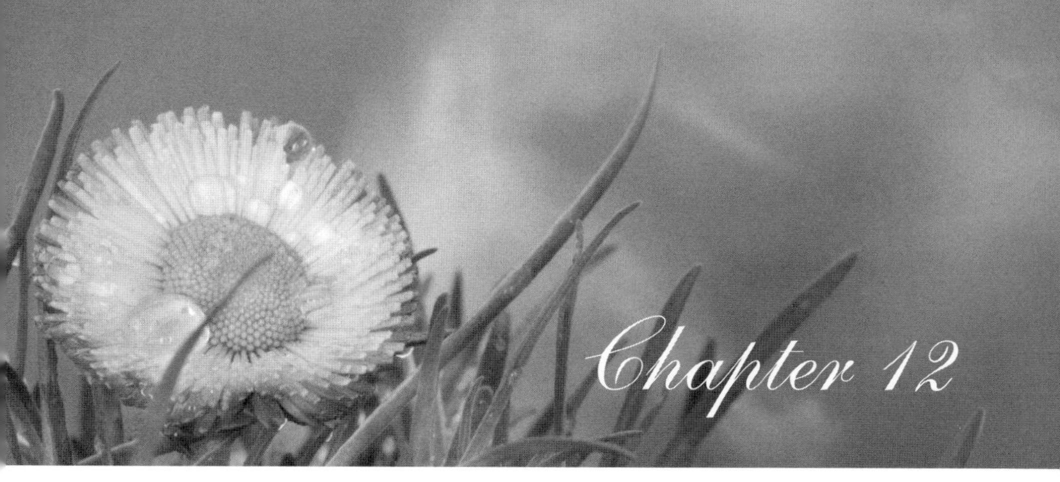

A Final Note

Taking Care

To care for the dying, we must embrace our humanity.

—Walter Hunter, M.D.

Burning Brightly, Burning Dimly

Caring for patients who are at the end of life is one of the most difficult, yet rewarding, experiences a nurse can have. It takes skill, wisdom, and courage to be present for the patient and for the patient's family at this crucial part of a person's life. You might experience the same doubts and fears that your patient does. You might find yourself agonizing over the questions about the meaning of life and hope. Sometimes working with a dying patient can remind you of your own personal losses. To be present for your patients, you must also take care of yourself.

The late Frank Lamendola, RN, Ph.D., a nurse leader in end-of-life care, identified how your energy and compassion can ebb and flow. He called it burning brightly, burning dimly (Lamendola, 1996). You are going to have those times when you feel you have given the best of yourself and your skills for the patient and the family. Those are the times of burning brightly. "You enter into the experience willingly and openly, not as a bystander, but as a participant in the lives of your patients and their families" (Lamendola, 1996, p.16R).

And you are definitely going to have the times of burning dimly. Those are the days when you're fatigued and find it hard to give compassionately of yourself. A hospice nurse said it well the day she reported to her supervisor, "I can't take one more sad story. I have no more tears left."

During those times when you burn dimly, step back and give yourself a breather. If you are feeling "worn out," consider ways to renew yourself. Some nurses use meditation, relaxation, exercise, or journaling. If you are struggling with the spiritual issues around meaning and existence, perhaps consider it as a good time to seek guidance from your own community of faith, a chaplain, or a trusted colleague. Also consider what you can do within your institution or agency. Some hospital units, long-term care facilities, or home health agencies have regular memorial services or staff retreats to remember patients and recognize the work you and other staff have done.

Living in the Present Moment

Just as every human being is unique, every dying experience is unique. You have the opportunity to experience remarkable spiritual and emotional fulfillment when your patient dies well. But, despite your best care and efforts, not all of your patients are going to die well. When you are a part of a difficult dying experience or a difficult death, avoid looking at it as a failure and second-guessing the care you have provided. A hospice nurse said of her first year of caring for dying patients, "I drove myself crazy when things didn't go well. I'd ask myself, 'What if I had upped the dose of morphine? Maybe I should have called the chaplain sooner. Why wasn't I there when the patient died?' I nearly burned out until a wiser, more experienced nurse took me aside and said, 'Look at the good things you did in that case. Give yourself credit and allow yourself to move on.'"

If you have an experience that does not go well or that drains you, take some time to reflect on it. What can you learn? How can this knowledge pave the way for the next patient? Consider this wisdom a gift. Then plant yourself firmly in the present for the patients you are caring for now and say, "I can do this, I am strong."

The Joy and the Laughter

Dr. Walter Hunter, a hospice medical director, says about working with the dying, "Laughter and joy can be a more effective medicine than anything we hope to produce in the laboratory" (Hamilton, 2001). Remember, those who are dying are also living, and laughter is a part of living.

Consider the story a hospice coordinator tells of a 67-year-old woman who was at home and nearing death. "I received a call from her very distraught son. He asked, 'When is Mom going to die?' I'd never met the patient, so I asked him some questions about her. He told me he was calling because his mother had gathered them to the bedside in the morning to tell them good-bye. 'But, she hasn't died yet, and I don't know if something is wrong.' I told him I'd have a nurse come out to visit and that I'd call him right away in the morning to see how things were going. The next day I called. He started to laugh when I asked how things were. 'Well,' he said, 'Mom gathered us all to the bedside again last night. She apologized for saying good-bye too soon. We didn't quite know what to say until she started to laugh and said, 'Of course, I've never done this before, so how would I know?' The son said it was a wonderful moment for the family. 'In all the worry about Mom dying, we'd forgotten how to laugh.' The patient died very peacefully two days later."

A Final Note

"Through the intimacy of caring, nurses also experience personal suffering and respond by seeking a balance of life and work and through deep personal reflection. This is the challenging and rewarding work of nursing" (Ferrell & Coyle, 2008, p.110.)

Caring for people at the end of life is the essence of nursing. We have the opportunity to witness and nurture the richness and grace of the human spirit in those final days and hours. Use this book to find out what you "don't know." Then use the resources listed to build something solid to stand upon so you can be present for your patients and families.

References

Ferrell, B.R. & Coyle, N. (2008). *The nature of suffering and the goals of nursing*. New York: Oxford University Press.

Hamilton, C. (2001). Caring for the seriously ill: 12 ethical imperatives for working with the dying. *Supportive Voice Newsletter of Supportive Care of the Dying* 7 (2): 4–5.

Lamendola, F. (1996). Keeping your compassion alive. *American Journal of Nursing* 96 (11): 16R-16T.

Index

Symbols

1997 Gallup poll, 24
6-month prognosis, hospice, 97

A

AAP (American Academy of Pediatrics), 84
ABC's of pain management, 25
acceptance of loss, grief, 70–72
acknowledgement
- grief, 73
- guiding patient/family through suffering, 54

active dying, 57–66
- children, 79
- clinical indicators, 58–62
- defined, 57–58
- resources, 66
- withdrawing life-sustaining treatment, 65

activities of daily living (ADLs), 7, 37
adjuvant medications, pain management, 28
adolescents, death of, 77
advance care planning, 11–21
- advance directives, 15, 19–20
- advocating for patients, 16–17
- barriers, 17–19
- courageous conversations, 11–12

cultural considerations, 20
DNR/DNI status, 16
elements of, 12–14
POLST forms, 16
resources, 22
advance directives, 15, 19–20
advocacy (as nursing role), xi, 4–5
accommodating family after death, 69–70
active dying communication, 63
advance care planning, 16–17
ensuring patients a holistic view, 52–53
hospice, 100
linking patient and medical system, 43–44
meeting needs of patient and family, 80–82, 107–108
Aging With Dignity Web site, 22
agonal breathing, 60
American Academy of Pediatrics (AAP), 84
American Nurses Association Code of Ethics, 111
anticonvulsants, 28
antidepressants, 28
antiolytics, dyspnea management, 38
anxiety, symptom management, 42
apnea, 60
artificial nutrition, ethical issues, 105
assessment
active dying, 58–62
care of dying children, 77–79
depression, 42–43
pain management, 25–27
physical symptoms, 36–43
suffering, 48–51
personal and family, 49–50
physical suffering, 48–49
spiritual suffering, 51
assumptions, cultural diversity, 89
autonomy, 104

B

barriers, advance care planning, 17–19
"Be Strong" clichés, 71
beneficence, 104
bereavement. *See* grief
bioethics. *See* ethical issues
body jerks, as indicator in active dying, 62
book resources, xii
cultural diversity, 93
grief, 74
pain management, 34
breathing changes, active dying, 60, 79
Byock, Dr. Ira, 50

C

Callanan, Maggie, 61
Caring Connections, 22
Cassel, Dr. Eric, 48
Chaplains, as members of health care team, 8
CHI (Children's Hospital International), 84
Child Life specialists, 80
children
death of, 75–83
active dying, 79
adult care *versus* child care, 76
assessment and intervention, 77–79
guiding children, 82–83
meeting needs of patient and family, 80–82
pain management, 78
resources, 84
symptoms, 79
loss and, 72

Children's Hospital International (CHI), 84
chronic illness, 2
City of Hope Web site, 34
clinical indicators, active dying, 58–62
clinical pain management, 27–28
communication
  active dying phase, 63
  dying children and their families, 80–82
  physicians and patients, 15
community resources, cultural diversity, 90
complementary therapies, pain management, 28–29
conflicts, ethical issues, 105–106
confusion, as indicator in active dying, 61
consciousness, as indicator in active dying, 61
constipation, symptom management, 39
corticosteroids, 28
Covinsky, K. E., 16
crisis, decision making and, 18–19
cultural diversity, 85–92
  advance care planning, 20
  advocating for patients/family, 91
  assumptions, 89
  community resources, 90
  ethical issues, 109
  listening to patients, 88
  medical interpreters, 89–90
  resources, 93
  stereotyping, 89
  understanding own beliefs, 87
cultural informants, 90
curative care, transition to palliative care, 6–7

D

death
  active dying, 57–66
    clinical indicators, 58–62
    defined, 57–58
  children, 75–83
    active dying, 79
    adult care *versus* child care, 76
    assessment and intervention, 77–79
    guiding children, 82–83
    meeting needs of patient and family, 80–82
    pain, 78
    resources, 84
    symptoms, 79
  grief, 67–73
    acceptance of loss, 70–72
    accommodating family needs, 69–70
    children and loss, 72
    nursing interventions after death, 68–69
    self care for the nurse, 73
death rattle, 60
decision making
  crisis and, 18–19
  ethical issues, 105–107
  nurse as guide, 108–109
delirium, as indicator in active dying, 61
depression, 42-43
developmental age, influence on dying children, 76
diarrhea, symptom management, 40
dieticians, as members of health care team, 8
dilemmas, ethical issues, 105–106
diminishing returns, pain management, 32
discomforts of hydration, 59

discounting clichés, 72
DNI (do not intubate) order, 16
DNR (do not resuscitate) order, 16
do not intubate (DNI) order, 16
do not resuscitate (DNR) order, 16
double effect principle, ethical issues, 105
durable health care powers of attorney, 15
dyspnea, symptom management, 37–38

E

elements of advance care planning, 12–14
emesis, symptom management, 40
End of Life/Palliative Education Resource Center (EPERC), 66
enemas, constipation management, 39
EPERC (End of Life/Palliative Education Resource Center), 66
ethical issues, 103–110
  culture and, 109
  decision making, 106–107
  dilemmas and conflicts, 105–106
  health care ethics, 104
  personal ethics/beliefs, 109
  resources, 111
euthanasia, 106

F

family
  engagement with pain management plan, 32
  preferences for care, 5
  suffering, 49–50
  support of patient goals/values, 14
fatigue
  as indicator in active dying, 58–59
  symptom management, 41
fears, pain management, 31–32
Final Gifts: Understanding the Special Awareness, Needs, and Communication of the Dying, 61
fluid intake, as indicator in active dying, 59
food intake, as indicator in active dying, 59
funeral rituals, 91

G

goals of patients, 13–14
grief, 67–73
  acceptance of loss, 70–72
  accommodating family needs, 69–70
  children and loss, 72
  nursing interventions after death, 68–69
  resources, 74
  self care for the nurse, 73
grimacing expressions, as indicator in active dying, 62
Growth House Web site, 74
guides (as nursing role), xi, 4–5
  active dying phase, 64–65
  assisting family to accept loss, 70–72
  decision making, 108–109
  guiding children through death, 82–83
  guiding patient/family through suffering, 53–54
  symptom management, 44–45
guiding principles, end of life care, 2–4

H

health care
- agents, 15, 20
- directives, 15
- ethics, 104
- powers of attorney, 15, 19
- proxies, 15
- team, 7–8

holistic view, suffering, 52–53
hope, advance care planning, 18
hospice, 3, 95–100
- 6-month prognosis, 97
- approaching families, 97–98
- Medicare benefit, 98–100
- philosophy of care, 95–96
- qualifications, 96–97
- resources, 101

Hospice and Palliative Nurse's Association (HPNA), 106
HPNA (Hospice and Palliative Nurse's Association), 106
Hunter, Dr. Walter, 115
hydration discomforts, 59

I

infants, death of, 76
inhalers, dyspnea management, 38
intake, as indicator in active dying, 59
integrative therapies
- as treatment for weight loss/loss of appetite, 40
- pain management, 28–29

Internet resources, xii
- active dying, 66
- Aging with Dignity Web site, 22
- Caring Connections, 22
- cultural diversity, 93
- death of children, 84
- grief, 74
- National Consensus Project for Quality End of Life Care, 10
- NHPCO, 10
- pain management, 34

involuntary body jerks, as indicator in active dying, 62

J

joy as effective medicine, 115
justice, 104

K

Kelley, Patricia, 61

L

Lamendola, Frank, RN, Ph.D., 113
laughter as effective medicine, 115
laxatives, constipation management, 39
levels of consciousness, as indicator in active dying, 61
life-extending treatment withdrawal, 65
life-sustaining treatment withdrawal, 65
listening skills
- guiding patient/family through suffering, 54
- pain management, 23–24

living wills, 15, 19
loss of appetite, symptom management, 40
lubricant stimulants, constipation management, 39

M

management
  pain, 23–33
    addressing fears, 31–32
    adjuvant medications, 28
    assessment, 25–27
    children, 78
    clinical pain management, 27–28
    integrative therapies, 28–29
    listening to the patient, 23–24
    meeting patient goals, 29–31
    resources, 33–34
  physical symptoms, 35–45
    anxiety, 42
    constipation, 39
    depression, 42
    diarrhea, 40
    dyspnea, 37–38
    fatigue, 41
    nausea and vomiting, 40
    skin disorders, 41
    weight loss/loss of appetite, 40
medical ethics. *See* ethical issues
medical interpreters, 89–90
medical system, linking patients to, 43–44
Medicare benefit, hospice, 98–100
medications, pain management, 28
moaning sounds, as indicator in active dying, 62

N

narcotic addiction, pain management, 31
National Consensus Project for Quality End of Life Care, 10
National Hospice and Palliative Care Organization (NHPCO), 3, 10
The Nature of Suffering, 48
nausea, symptom management, 40
nearing death awareness, 61
nebulizers, dyspnea management, 38
NHPCO (National Hospice and Palliative Care Organization), 3, 10
nonmaleficence, 104
nonpharmacy intervention. *See* integrative therapies
nonsteroidal anti-inflammatory drugs (NSAIDS), 28
NSAIDS (nonsteroidal anti-inflammatory drugs), 28
nursing roles, xi, 4–5
  advocacy
    accommodating family after death, 69–70
    active dying communication, 63
    advance care planning, 16–17
    assuring patients a holistic view, 52–53
    hospice, 100
    linking patient and medical system, 43–44
    meeting needs of patient and family, 80–82, 107–108
  guides
    active dying phase, 64–65
    advance care planning, 17–19
    assisting family to accept loss, 70–72
    decision making, 108–109
    guiding children through death, 82–83
    guiding patient/family through suffering, 53–54
    symptom management, 44–45
  skilled clinicians
    advance care planning, 12–15
    ethical decision making, 106–107
    understanding grief, 68–69

O

Office of Minority Health Resource Center (OMHRC), 93
OMHRC (Office of Minority Health Resource Center), 93
Oncology Nursing Society Multicultural Toolkits, 93
opioids, dyspnea management, 38
osmotic laxatives, constipation management, 39
output, as indicator in active dying, 61–62
oxygen delivery, dyspnea management, 38

P

pain management, 23–33
  addressing fears, 31–32
  adjuvant medications, 28
  assessment, 25–27
  children, 78
  clinical pain management, 27–28
  integrative therapies, 28–29
  listening to the patient, 23–24
  meeting patient goals, 29–31
  resources, 33–34
palliative care
  defined, 2–3
  transition from curative care, 6–7
patients
  engagement with pain management plan, 32
  experiences with death, 14
  goals and values, 13–14
  linking to medical system, 43–44
  preferences for care, 5, 54
  understanding of illness, 14
personal suffering, 49–50
pharmacists, as members of health care team, 8
philosophy of care, hospice, 95–96
physical suffering, 48–49
physical symptom management, 35–45
  anxiety, 42
  constipation, 39
  depression, 42
  diarrhea, 40
  dyspnea, 37–38
  fatigue, 41
  nausea and vomiting, 40
  skin disorders, 41
  weight loss/loss of appetite, 40
physician aid in dying, ethical issues, 106
Physician's Order for Life-Sustaining Treatment (POLST) forms, 16
physician-assisted suicide, ethical issues, 106
physicians
  as member of health care team, 7
  communication with patients, 15
  responsibilities with advance care planning, 18
"picking" behavior, 62
POLST (Physician's Order for Life-Sustaining Treatment) forms, 16
powers of attorney, 15, 19
preferences of patients, 5, 54
preschoolers, death of, 77
presence, 53
pressure ulcers, 41
principles
  clinical pain management, 27–28
  end of life care, 2–4
pruritus, 41

Q

qualifications for hospice, 96–97

R

religious clichés, 72
resources, xii, 10
  active dying, 66
  advance care planning, 15, 22
  cultural diversity, 90, 93
  death of children, 84
  ethical issues, 111
  grief, 74
  hospice, 101
  pain management, 33–34
  physical symptom management, 46
resuscitation, ethical issues, 105
rites (funerals), 91
rituals (funerals), 91
roles (nursing), xi, 4–5
  advocacy
    accommodating family after death, 69–70
    active dying communication, 63
    advance care planning, 16–17
    assuring patients a holistic view, 52–53
    hospice, 100
    linking patient and medical system, 43–44
    meeting needs of patient and family, 80–82, 107–108
  guides
    active dying phase, 64–65
    advance care planning, 17–19
    assisting family to accept loss, 70–72
    decision making, 108–109
    guiding children through death, 82–83
    guiding patient/family through suffering, 53–54
    symptom management, 44–45
  skilled clinicians
    advance care planning, 12–15
    ethical decision making, 106–107
    understanding grief, 68–69

S

school age children, death of, 77
self care for nurses, 73, 113–114
shortness of breath (SOB). *See* dyspnea
skilled clinicians (as nursing role), xi, 4–5
  advance care planning, 12–15
  ethical decision making, 106–107
  understanding grief, 68–69
skin color changes, as indicator in active dying, 60–61
skin disorders, symptom management, 41
sleep changes, active dying, 79
SOB (shortness of breath). *See* dyspnea
social workers, as members of health care team, 8
sphincter control, as indicator in active dying, 61–62
spiritual care workers, as members of health care team, 8
spiritual suffering, 51
stereotyping, cultural diversity, 89
stimulant laxatives, constipation management, 39
stool softeners, constipation management, 39

suffering, 47–55
  assessment, 48–51
    personal and family, 49–50
    physical suffering, 48–49
    spiritual suffering, 51
  holistic view, 52–53
supportive phrases, advance care planning, 17
symptoms
  death of children, 79
  physical symptom management, 35–45
    anxiety, 42
    depression, 42
    diarrhea, 40
    dyspnea, 37–38
    fatigue, 41
    nausea and vomiting, 40
    skin disorders, 41
    weight loss/loss of appetite, 40

T

team approach, 7–8
temperature changes, active dying, 79
terminal delirium, nearing death awareness, 61
toddlers, death of, 76
topical therapies, 28
touch
  guiding patient/family through suffering, 54
  respect of patient wishes, 88
transition (curative care to palliative care), 6–7

U

understanding of illness (patient perspective), 14
urine output, as indicator in active dying, 61–62

V

values, patients, 13–14
ventilator support, ethical issues, 105
vomiting, symptom management, 40

W-Z

weakness, as indicator in active dying, 58–59
Web resources, xii
  active dying, 66
  Aging with Dignity Web site, 22
  Caring Connections, 22
  cultural diversity, 93
  death of children, 84
  grief, 74
  National Consensus Project for Quality End of Life Care, 10
  NHPCO, 10
  pain management, 34
weight loss, symptom management, 40
WHO (World Health Organization), principles of clinical pain management, 27
wills, 19
withdrawing life-sustaining treatment, 65
World Health Organization (WHO), principles of clinical pain management, 27

Books Published by the Honor Society of Nursing, Sigma Theta Tau International

To Comfort Always: A Nurse's Guide to End of Life Care, Linda Norlander, 2008.

Ready, Set, Go Lead! A Primer for Emerging Health Care Leaders, Dickenson-Hazard, 2008.

Words of Wisdom From Pivotal Nurse Leaders, Houser and Player, 2008.

Tales From The Pager Chronicles, Rancour, 2008.

The Nurse's Etiquette Advantage, Pagana, 2008.

NURSE: A World of Care, Jaret, 2008. Published by Emory University and distributed by the Honor Society of Nursing, Sigma Theta Tau International.

Johns Hopkins Nursing Evidence-Based Practice Model and Guidelines, Newhouse, Dearholt, Poe, Pugh, and White, 2007.

Nursing Without Borders: Values, Wisdom, Success Markers, Weinstein and Brooks, 2007.

Synergy: The Unique Relationship Between Nurses and Patients, Curley, 2007.

Conversations With Leaders: Frank Talk From Nurses (and Others) on the Front Lines of Leadership, Hansen-Turton, Sherman, and Ferguson, 2007.

Pivotal Moments in Nursing: Leaders Who Changed the Path of a Profession, Houser and Player, 2004 (Volume I) and 2007 (Volume II).

Shared Legacy, Shared Vision: The W.K. Kellogg Foundation and the Nursing Profession, Lynaugh, Smith, Grace, Sena, de Villalobos, and Hlalele, 2007.

Daily Miracles: Stories and Practices of Humanity and Excellence in Health Care, Briskin and Boller, 2006.

A Daybook for Nurse Leaders and Mentors. Sigma Theta Tau International, 2006.

When Parents Say No: Religious and Cultural Influences on Pediatric Healthcare Treatment, Linnard-Palmer, 2006.

Healthy Places, Healthy People: A Handbook for Culturally Competent Community Nursing Practice, Dreher, Shapiro, and Asselin, 2006.

The HeART of Nursing: Expressions of Creative Art in Nursing, Second Edition, Wendler, 2005.

Making a Difference: Stories from the Point of Care, volumes I & II, Hudacek, 2005.

A Daybook for Nurses: Making a Difference Each Day, Hudacek, 2004.

Ordinary People, Extraordinary Lives: The Stories of Nurses, Smeltzer and Vlasses, 2003.

The Language of Nursing Theory and Metatheory, King and Fawcett, 1997.